Praise for Sacred Massage

"Touch can be a very sacred thing when shared by two individuals with an intent that is aligned. Debra has a wonderful gift for sharing a touch modality that will engender a greater heart connection between you and those you decide to connect with on this level.…She deftly provides a simple, yet powerful, roadmap for sacred massage that can reach deep into your soul and that of your loved ones."

—DB McPeek, Reiki master

"Debra DeAngelo makes it clear how and why massage is a key to healthy living and connection. As a professional massage therapist, DeAngelo has literal hands-on experience on how important touch is to healing and health and that comes through in the pages of *Sacred Massage*, but she doesn't stop there. DeAngelo goes deeper into the practice of massage sharing important components and how to take your personal touch practice to the next level. As a former massage therapist, I found her book to be a beautiful balance of practical massage tips and spiritual depth."

—Phoenix LeFae, author of *Walking in Beauty*

"This book is a gift for the soul that will allow you to experience a lightness of spirit, allowing you to attract amazing things into your world. I cannot express how vital this book is because the imprints of our past stored in the body can be freed to make room for a beautiful and intuitive future. You will grasp the power of using massage as a path to awakening happiness with this magnificently fun compilation."

—Shannon Yrizarry, author of *Kundalini Energy*

"With emotional intelligence and expert physical skill, Debra helped unwind the chronic knots in my back and neck. Getting a massage every week has reduced my chronic pain and improved my quality of life. Reading her book might be the first step in that direction for you or someone you love."

—Sandra Aamodt, author of *Welcome to Your Brain*

"I've spent years playing hit or miss in an attempt to soothe my constant feelings of fear and worry. With massage, I finally found my solace. The massage table became a sanctuary, where the gentle feeling of hands on my skin told my mind and body, 'Relax. Breathe. You are safe in this moment.'"

—Kimberley Tufveson, massage client

"This thoughtful and gracious book contains ample information for the laity to practice sacred touch and magical massage on their loved ones. The author includes the perfect balance of professional and relatable guidance, providing full instruction in such a way that the reader does not feel intimidated or overwhelmed. The book provides complete explanations of massage and touch techniques that even the most inexperienced practitioner can easily implement. Additionally, the divine component of interlacing massage with magical practice deepens the healing potential. ... This book is a gift."

—Katrina Rasbold, witch, Reiki master, and author of *Uncrossing*

"*Sacred Massage* arrives as an antidote to touch starvation, a call to remember that intentional touch can offer healing and restoration. The magic of touch and the impact of skin-on-skin contact is more than physiological and beyond the list of benefits to the body; this book reminds us, encourages us, and inspires us to offer loving care to our worn bodies as part of a ritual practice. Inviting the sacred into our lives can begin with remembering we hold this magic in our hands and can offer it to ourselves and others."

—Irisanya Moon, author of *Practically Pagan: An Alternative Guide to Health & Well-Being*

Sacred MASSAGE

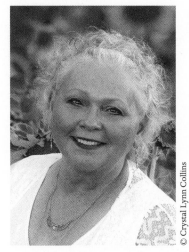

About the Author

Debra DeAngelo has been a certified massage practitioner for more than twenty years. She runs her own private practice where she incorporates spiritual techniques into every session. In addition to developing her own method called "Blended Deep Swedish Massage," Debra is certified in hot stone, Ayurvedic, reflexology, Reiki, and other massage styles. She also writes feature stories and book reviews for *SageWoman* and *Witches & Pagans* magazines.

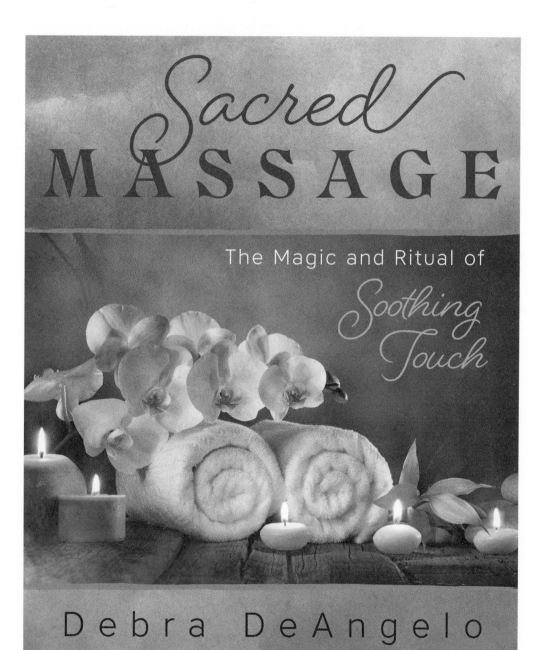

Sacred
MASSAGE

The Magic and Ritual of

Soothing Touch

Debra DeAngelo

Llewellyn Publications
Woodbury, Minnesota

FIRST EDITION
First Printing, 2023

Book design by R. Brasington
Cover design by Kevin R. Brown
Editing by Marjorie Otto

Interior Illustrations:
Mary Ann Zapalac: 160, 166, 170, 173, 176, 178, 180, 187, 189, 191, 194, 196, 198, 202, 204, 206, 211, 245–257
Llewellyn Art Department: 65, 125, 129, 144–150, 156

Llewellyn Publications is a registered trademark of Llewellyn Worldwide Ltd.

Library of Congress Cataloging-in-Publication Data (Pending)
ISBN: 978-0-7387-7267-7

Llewellyn Worldwide Ltd. does not participate in, endorse, or have any authority or responsibility concerning private business transactions between our authors and the public.

   All mail addressed to the author is forwarded, but the publisher cannot, unless specifically instructed by the author, give out an address or phone number.

   Any internet references contained in this work are current at publication time, but the publisher cannot guarantee that a specific location will continue to be maintained. Please refer to the publisher's website for links to authors' websites and other sources.

Llewellyn Publications
A Division of Llewellyn Worldwide Ltd.
2143 Wooddale Drive
Woodbury, MN 55125-2989
www.llewellyn.com

Printed in the United States of America

Other Books by Debra DeAngelo

The Elements of Horse Spirit (2020)
Pagan Curious (2022)

Dedication

This book is dedicated to my Magical Mother Midwives: Aradia, Athena, Bastet, Brigid, Danu, Diana, Gaia, Hygieia, Iris, Isis, White Tara, and most especially, Kuan Yin.

With Appreciation

Sincere gratitude to my amazing editor, Angela Wix, for all the encouragement and validation, and for guiding me toward polishing this little gem until it shined. Thank you for believing in me.

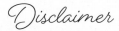

Disclaimer

The information contained in this book is for educational purposes only, and is not intended or implied to be a substitute for professional medical advice, diagnosis, or treatment. Readers are advised to consult a medical professional or healthcare provider before proceeding with these practices, in particular, those with a history of health issues.

You assume full responsibility for how you choose to use the information in this book. Neither this publisher nor the author may be held liable for any issue or injury associated with information in this book.

Completion of this book and mastery of its practices does not connote any sort of professional certification or licensing, nor does it allow you to accept payment for your services in any form. Presenting yourself as a massage therapist or practitioner without the required licensing for your location is against the law.

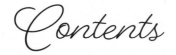

Contents

Activities—xiv

Illustrations—xv

Cheat Sheets—xvii

Foreword—xix

Introduction—1

Part One: Before You Begin

Chapter One: The Language of Touch—9

Chapter Two: What You'll Need—31

Chapter Three: Concerns, Contraindications, and
    Assorted Miscellanea—43

Part Two: The Spiritual and Magical Side of Massage

Chapter Four: Touch Is Spiritual—63

Chapter Five: Let's Make Magic—85

Chapter Six: Touch Is Magical—111

Part Three: The Practice of Soothing Touch

Chapter Seven: The Tools and Techniques of Touch—135

Chapter Eight: Touching the Back of the Body—153

Chapter Nine: Touching the Front of the Body—185

Chapter Ten: Bringing It All Together in Sacred Massage—215

Conclusion: You Have Everything You Need—239

Resources—241

Appendix: Cheat Sheets—245

Bibliography—259

Activities

Meditation for Embracing Love and Compassion—19

Meditation for Directing Love and Compassion—20

Practicing Thoughtful Touch—22

Inviting Deity into Massage—66

Developing a Divine Relationship (Meditation, Prayer, Study)—67

Cleansing and Dedicating Your Massage Space—89

Cleansing and Dedicating Your Magical Massage Table—92

Create an Altar—108

Grounding and Centering Meditation—115

Imagine Grounding and Centering—116

Imagine Inviting Divine Energy and Deity—119

Feel the Energy in Your Hands—125

Meditation for Energizing Your Hands—126

Finding and Clearing the Chakras—131

Exploring Your Hands Anew—135

Techniques of Touch—137

Getting to Know Your Tools—143

Ritual to Cleanse and Dedicate Your Healing Hands—215

"Just Spread the Oil" Sequences—217

Full-Body Massage Routine—220

Illustrations

Figure 1: Cho Ku Rei Symbol—65

Figure 2: Hamsa and Nazar—125

Figure 3: Chakra Figure—129

Figure 4: Duckbill Massage Technique—144

Figure 5: Iron Massage Technique—145

Figure 6: Paintbrush Massage Technique—146

Figure 7: Powerpoint Massage Technique—146

Figure 8: Rake Massage Technique—147

Figure 9: Scraper Massage Technique—148

Figure 10: Snowplow Massage Technique—149

Figure 11: Steamroller Massage Technique—150

Figure 12: Lateral vs. Medial—156

Figure 13: Back, Spine, and Muscles—160

Figure 14: Back of Shoulders, Scapula, and Neck—166

Figure 15: Back of Neck—170

Figure 16: Bottom of Foot/Sole—173

Figure 17: Back of Calf—176

Figure 18: Back of Thigh—178

Figure 19: Glutes—180

Figure 20: Top of Foot—187

Figure 21: Front Lower Leg—189

Figure 22: Front of Thigh—191

Figure 23: Stomach—194

Figure 24: Hand—196

Figure 25: Lower Arm—198

Figure 26: Upper Arm—198

Figure 27: Pectorals—202

Figure 28: Front of Shoulder—204

Figure 29: Front of Neck—206

Figure 30: Jaw and Scalp—211

Cheat Sheets

Arm—201

Back—165

Back of the Neck—171

Calf—177

Foot (Bottom)—174

Foot (Top)—188

Front of Lower Leg—190

Glutes—183

Hand—197

Jaw / Face—213

Neck—208

Pectorals and Shoulders—20

Scalp and Ears—210

Shoulders and Scapula—169

Stomach—195

Thigh (Back)—179

Thigh (Front)—193

Foreword

I know this book is about massage, but Debra really gets so much deeper on themes I think, in today's times, are vital.

We need to care for each other with genuine intent and compassion to rise from the ashes. Without going too far on a tangent, I find this very connected to themes in our society that are truly suffering without this intent.

Education and healthcare are truly suffering. They have been decimated with a lack of focus and forgetting to truly care for people. Our society has become so caught up in the ridiculous pursuit of box-checking we have lost our connection to human kindness and what really matters.

Debra gets that. It does not matter how you get there, just try. Just be there for each other. Have an intention and a plan to show those around you that you care about them. Care enough to know them, find what they need, and adjust accordingly to what works both for you and for those you care about.

I hear this frequently from patients when they see a doctor: "They didn't even touch me." This is important to people. Touch is a connection, human to human, and is necessary.

I love everything about how Debra seeks to make her massage space healing and welcoming. She reaches out to the universe to connect not only to our earthly beings but to things not always acknowledged: nature, cosmos, religion—I don't care what you call it. It is around us and can be harnessed to create a space of love and connection.

Teaching is a place where the term "differentiation" is used. This means tailoring what you do to the person in front of you. This is how I try to practice. Everyone has different needs, and even that changes over time. In writing this book, Debra aims to teach you how to connect with a loved one to help them heal and attain peace.

I will take from this book a continued quest to be the best I can be to others. I will continue to wear my healing hand pendant and think of Debra and her gifts. I hope you can too. We all need each other to prosper on this earth journey.

I have been blessed to be a client of Debra's and, truly, I always leave from a session with her feeling lighter, warmer, and able to spread more kindness out after bringing so much in. We all can manifest this every day for each other. We can create altars and find music and spread beautiful scents all around us. This will bring us all to the ground to be whole.

Karen Mo, MD
UC Davis family physician

Introduction

I didn't set out to be a massage therapist. Like life, it just happened while I was busy making other plans. I'll blame serendipity.

I was working as the editor of my little community newspaper and needed to supplement my income when I'd reached the irrefutable conclusion that the only way to save my own life was to untangle myself from my miserable first marriage and move forward as a solo act. But I needed more money than what a small-town newspaper editor makes to pay the bills. After an eight-hour day saturated in writing, reading, reporting, and editing, the last thing I wanted to do was more of the same. I needed a second job and income that didn't involve sitting at a keyboard and staring at a computer monitor.

But what?

With two children to support and bills tapping their feet waiting to be paid, I didn't have the luxury of taking my sweet time exploring supplemental careers. Pondering this pressing dilemma, I flashed on a news story I'd written a few years prior about a local massage therapist. As part of the story, I received a massage—my first. After nearly a decade of hunching over a keyboard, my neck, shoulders, and back were one chronically clenched fist of stress and strain. That massage was pure, astonishing heaven. I remembered that exquisite relief, and thought, "Why not massage?" Massage is the polar opposite of journalism in every way. Journalism is intellectually focused, objective, emotionally detached, sedentary, high stress, and combative. Massage is emotionally focused, interpersonal, physically active, nurturing, low stress, compassionate, peaceful, and quiet. Massage gave me access to a box of tools I hadn't had much opportunity to use in journalism. Massage allowed me to exhale.

Besides serving as a counterpoint to journalism, as well as a pretty respectable income (about four times more per hour than my editor paycheck), learning to do massage was emotionally enriching and downright magical. Massage schooling isn't just about doing—it's also about receiving. We learned the techniques by practicing on each other. Let me tell you, as a lifelong touch-starved, touch-aversive person, I got hooked on touch in a snap. Experiencing compassionate, nurturing touch for the first time in my life—as well as learning to give it—was transformational. I discovered a side of myself I didn't even know was there: healer.

I grew up in a dysfunctional, alcoholic household, where physical contact was practically nonexistent. Just a simple hug or kiss was a rare occurrence. And compassion? Soothing touch? What are those? I was touch-starved all through my childhood and on into high school—until I discovered boys and sex. It was worth all that clumsy teenage fumbling for the holding and cuddling that came afterward. Some might view that as "promiscuity," but they're way off base. Sex was never the main attraction. It was the gentle holding that came afterward.

In college, studying psychology, I learned an interesting term: *skin hunger*. Bingo. That was the term for the soul ache that had permeated my entire life. I didn't come from a loving, demonstrative family, even without the alcoholism. My mother didn't kiss or cuddle us, and on the rare occasions she held me, there was no more emotional connection involved than holding a sack of flour. My father did somewhat better—he'd ask for a hug and kiss goodnight. Just in case one of us died in our sleep and never saw each other again. Well then … on that note, sweet dreams, kiddo.

Not until I had children of my own did I experience the peace and warmth of close, loving touch. My babies were excellent teachers and provided all my on-the-job training about the value of touch. The relaxed, trusting warmth and weight of a sleeping baby against your chest, right beside your heart, is immersion therapy on how loving touch feels: complete safety, complete trust. My babies taught me that I was a natural hugger and holder all along, but never had an opportunity to express those skills. Now, I'm a master! I love warm, squishy, full-body hugs, and I love people who can return them even more. Touch just feels *good*—even if it takes a while for you to learn that.

I bring up my touch-deprived early life to show that even if you're uncomfortable touching others or being touched by them, be open to the possibility that this can change. As you learn to fuel your touch with heartfelt compassion, you may also discover that not only are you good at it, but you also really like it—both giving and receiving. You can get a head start on that learning process by getting a massage yourself. A lot of them, in fact! You'll not only discover the healing power of touch, but you'll also get some exposure to the feel and pace of a massage and learn what you like and what you don't. And besides, as you learn massage techniques yourself in this book, you'll have a perfect excuse to "indulge" in getting massage. It's all research!

Learning to Touch

The ink on my signature for my divorce papers was barely dry when I enrolled in massage school and started exploring what giving *and* receiving massage felt like. A whole new world opened up to me, internally and externally. When I graduated, I knew lots of techniques for providing relief and relaxation, but I was still just a pup. Our teacher told us on graduation day that although we'd mastered the basic skills and could legally call ourselves massage practitioners, we wouldn't be *great* massage therapists until at least a hundred bodies had passed under our hands. We had plenty of schooling and practice, but true mastery comes from lots and lots of *doing*: massaging all sorts of bodies—young, old, thick, thin, athletic, sedentary—all with a lot in common, but each one entirely unique. Working on people isn't like working on cars. Cars are interchangeable; people aren't. You can't just do your same massage routine on each person the same way and call it a day. No, you must adjust and customize your touch for each patient. The best way to learn how to do that is by doing it.

In this book, we'll learn by doing. This book doesn't substitute for massage schooling. It won't earn you any certificate or title or allow you to present yourself as a professional massage therapist, but you will have lots of experience for providing relaxing, soothing, healing, loving massage to a loved one, relative, partner, child, or friend. We'll learn many of the basic techniques and approaches I learned in massage school, but we'll also learn what I *didn't* learn in massage school: how to infuse a massage with divine compassion and love, as well as how to approach a massage session as a magical healing ritual.

There's much more to massage than knowing the terrain of a human body and how to spread oil over it and press here and push there. That's the physical part of massage. There's also a spiritual, magical side to massage, and with those skills, we'll elevate a typical massage experience into a comprehensive sacred, magical experience—Sacred Massage. It's all about the touch—specifically, the quality of the touch and who is providing it. Think about the most loving, gentle touch you've ever known—maybe a parent, grandparent, or spouse. Did you immediately relax with that touch—maybe from a warm hand on your back or shoulder—and feel safe and loved? That kind of touch comes not from the hands, but from the heart. That's where the energy begins. Besides learning the physical tools and techniques of massage, we'll open up to the warm, compassionate love in your own heart, and learn to channel it right through your hands—with a little divine participation, of course, and a little sprinkle of magic.

What I Bring to the (Massage) Table

In addition to my basic massage practitioner certificate (with a focus in Swedish massage), I've taken continuing education in Reiki, polarity therapy, deep tissue, deep tissue for ilio-psoas, hot stone massage, assisted stretching and joint mobilization, Ayurveda, foot reflexology, pathology for massage therapy, massage therapy for PTSD, facial massage, and aromatherapy. I started my own private massage practice in 2001 and have a home office. Following my retirement from journalism in 2018, I've focused exclusively on massage. (And writing books!)

I've cherry-picked from these modalities to craft my own moves, techniques, and style, which I loosely describe as "Deep Swedish." However, that's just the physical side of it. My spiritual approach to massage springs from my roots in the Pagan community, where a universe of spiritual and magical traditions coexist, along with deities and practices from a variety of cultures. I discovered the Pagan community about the same time I enrolled in massage school, so my massage and magical skills developed side by side. I've discovered that magic and massage dovetail quite nicely.

Using the techniques in this book, I'll share a variety of techniques for relieving tension, stress, and soreness, as well as guidance for connecting to your own heart and divine spirit, and channeling that energy into a spiritual, magical massage experience. Your soothing hands, your loving heart, and your divine spirit are the foundation of Sacred Massage. Everything else is just technique.

If you don't have any massage experience at all and are concerned that that you don't have the skills or aptitude for becoming a healer, let me reassure you: You most certainly do. The fact that you picked this book up confirms that you're ready, willing, and able to embrace the loving, healing art of Sacred Massage. You already have what it takes. I'm just going to show you what's already there. Borrowing from the Sanskrit term "Namaste," which means "The divine in me honors the divine in you," the divine in me already sees the divine in you. You just need to see it too.

How We'll Proceed

This book is divided into three parts. In the first, Before You Begin, you'll learn to view touch in a new way—as a form of nonverbal communication and connection, and how touch soothes and heals. You'll also get a heads-up on the items and supplies you'll need to get started, as well as various concerns to take into consideration before doing massage on your loved one. The second part, The Spiritual and Magical Side of Massage, is your introduction to everything they *don't* teach you in massage school: infusing your massage work with divine healing energy, and taking a magical approach to massage.

We'll go "hands on" in the third part, The Practice of Soothing Touch, and learn all the skills and techniques your hands are capable of, as well as how to use these techniques on each area of the body, step by step. And yes, in part three, we will be putting everything we're learning to use: we'll be doing actual massage one area of the body at a time, and, finally, learning not only to meld it into one complete full-body massage, but also how to transform that regular massage into a Sacred Massage.

In the third part, we'll be creating a notebook of "cheat sheets" for each area as we learn. You'll have a much easier time learning, practicing, and mastering the techniques for these areas by writing them down in your cheat sheet notebook as we go. You'll use that notebook as a guide while you actually practice the techniques.

The cheat sheets are listed alphabetically after the main table of contents, and there is an appendix of all the cheat sheets at the end of the book, in the order they're done in a massage. You could use the appendix as is instead of a notebook; however, be aware that the paper will get oily as you practice, so your book will likely become an ooey, gooey, oily mess. You could tear the appendix pages out and use them as your cheat sheets as you practice; however, if you're like me and the thought of dismembering or mutilating a book horrifies you, you'll be much happier creating your own notebook.

All Those Activities

As we go along, you'll notice "Activity" in the subsection headlines. "Activity" doesn't mean "keep reading," it means "stop and practice this." Some activities are meditations, some are rituals, and others are things for you to practice, either on yourself or your practice partner. It's important to actually *do* these things rather than just read through them, because massage is a kinesthetic learning process. Learning by doing also provides another avenue for your brain to soak up all this new information. It's kind of like cooking: There's a big difference between reading through a recipe and actually making it. If all you ever do is read the recipes, you'll never learn to cook.

There is a table of contents for the activities listed after the main table of contents so you can easily return to any activity you wish to practice or repeat.

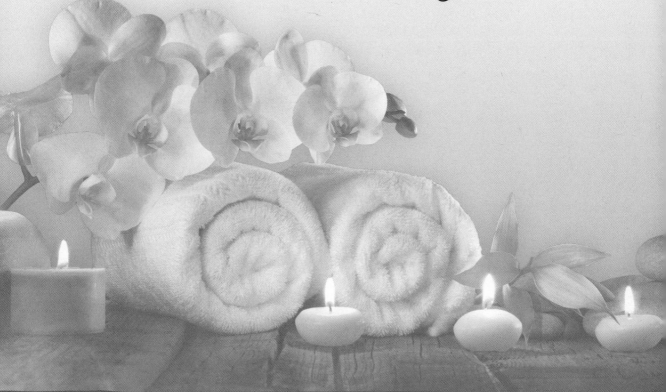

PART ONE

Before You Begin

Chapter 1

The Language of Touch

Music is often called "the universal language," but another language easily surpasses it: touch. True, music is part of all human cultures worldwide, but so is touch. However, touch has one up on music: It's spoken across, and between, species. All living things understand it, within their own species and without. When dogs lick each other's faces or horses stand nose to tail rhythmically nipping each other's backs, they're communicating. They're speaking the language of touch. People and animals can have entire conversations through touch without ever uttering a word. Gently stroke your pet's fur and watch the "reply" in their face or body language. Even plants speak this universal language, through their branches and roots, sometimes assisted by a complex subterranean network of fungus called mycelium. Sometimes, the communication is obvious, like hugging, kissing, petting, and scratching, but it can also be very subtle. Just cuddling next to another person or holding hands can lower blood pressure and induce a feeling of safety and serenity.

Touch is the first communication we receive just after birth—it's our true primary language. Our caretakers hold us close and touch our faces and hands. We open our eyes for the first time to gaze upon their face and into their eyes, and a loving bond unlike any other begins to blossom. Many mammals immediately lick their newborns, not only cleaning them, but increasing blood circulation. They literally begin their lives with massage! The olfactory bond is so strong from these early moments that the mothers will risk their lives and fight to the death to fiercely protect those babies. We humans have a lot to learn from animals, and are catching on to the importance of immediate physical contact between mother and infant. It's now common practice to place a fresh, wet, squalling newborn directly onto a mother's bare chest. Most newborns immediately calm down when they feel the warm comfort of Mama's skin and recognize the rhythm of her heartbeat and breathing.

They recognize her voice, and open their eyes, and look around at this strange new world for the first time.

Long before there were words much beyond grunts, growls, and whoops, stretching back more than five million years to our common ancestor with the apes, we communicated with facial expression, posture, and touch. From gentle co-grooming to shoving to biting in an attack, each type of touch was a clear communication: *I like you; Get out of my way; I'm angry.* Our DNA (and the DNA of all species) is hardwired to innately understand and communicate with touch.

Consider how much you can communicate through touch with just your index finger: a poke in the ribs; a tap on the shoulder; a touch of a teardrop; a long, slow, luscious drag down the spine. Even if you didn't speak the same language, the other person would understand your message loud and clear: *Hey! Excuse me; What's wrong? You turn me on.*

Massage also speaks the language of touch; however, the communication is mostly one way and narrower in scope. When we "speak" to another person through massage, we're saying, *I care about you. You matter to me. I want to relieve your pain. I want to relieve your anxiety. I want you to feel better. I want you to relax.* And, most of all, we're reassuring them, *You are safe here.*

Sacred Massage transports us back to our mother's arms. We feel completely safe and secure. We melt into the warmth and security of those strong, loving arms, confident that nothing bad can happen to us here. "Sleeping like a baby" really *is* a thing. Babies sleep peacefully and soundly, completely limp and relaxed, without anxieties or thoughts running through their minds—particularly when being lovingly rocked by a parent or caretaker. A guardian's watchful presence instills complete relaxation in us because we feel so very safe and loved. In Sacred Massage, we seek to recreate that experience: complete safety, complete trust, complete peace, complete relaxation. We communicate this without uttering a word. Our hands do all the talking.

Touch Is Necessary

Touch does much more than communicate. There's more to touch than just touch. It facilitates healing, both physically and psychologically. During a massage, a person can relax and sink into a calm and open state where they're receptive to healing energy. As for the massage therapist, there's a lot more going on than just covering the skin with oil and squeezing on some tight muscles. In addition to the physical massage techniques, there's an intention for healing and an overall sense of compassion, peace, and goodwill.

Respected organizations such as the Mayo Clinic and National Center for Complementary and Integrative Health have conducted research that validate massage as a healing catalyst for a variety of conditions, both physical and psychological.[1]

Although some view massage as frivolous pampering (which may be true of what some of us in the biz call "fluff and buff" for top dollar at a fancy spa or resort—however, a little pleasure and pampering never hurt anybody!), therapeutic massage is coming into mainstream acceptance as a component for good health, even amongst the toughest critics: the medical and science communities.[2,3] Even very light touch or energy-only modalities are gaining acceptance as skeptics must admit that something positive is going on.

In India, regular massage is accepted as a crucial part of maintaining good health.[4] Frequent massage is part of the culture, and not viewed as an extravagance, but rather, a part of all the components of good health, just like sleep, exercise, and good nutrition. The western world has some catching up to do in how it views the value of massage. Massage is necessary! What a different world it would be if everyone got regular massage, and reconnected to their own bodies and spirits, and let go of their stress! Now, sure, frequent massage is financially out of reach for most people—but not for those who know how to massage each other or who have a loved one who can provide it. By the time you finish this book, that will be *you*! To be clear, "too much massage" is not a thing. You could give—and receive—massage every day if you wanted to. Call me a dreamer, but if it was *my* perfect world, massage would be as much a part of each day as eating or sleeping.

Regular (let alone daily) professional massage therapy, although optimal for physical and psychological health, can be impractical or even impossible for several reasons. First and foremost, at $80 per hour and more, the cost of regular physical massage adds up quickly. For many people, the ongoing cost is prohibitive. Another barrier to getting massage is mobility, such as when a person cannot move or be moved easily. Distance can also

---

1. Mayo Clinic Staff, "Massage: Get In Touch with Its Many Benefits," Mayo Clinic, accessed July 15, 2022, https://www.mayoclinic.org/healthy-lifestyle/stress-management/in-depth/massage/art-20045743; National Center for Complementary and Integrative Health, "Massage Therapy: What You Need to Know," accessed July 15, 2022, https://www.nccih.nih.gov/health/massage-therapy-what-you-need-to-know.

2. Markham Heid, "The Science-Backed Benefits of Massage," Elemental, June 6, 2019. https://elemental.medium.com/the-science-backed-benefits-of-massage-6d1a198c67a5.

3. Florida Academy, "The Science Behind Massage Therapy," Florida Academy.edu, August 13, 2019, https://florida-academy.edu/science-behind-massage-therapy/.

4. Nona Walla, "Why You Need a Daily Massage," ETimes/Times of India.com, March 10, 2019, https://timesofindia.indiatimes.com/life-style/health-fitness/de-stress/why-you-need-a-daily-massage/articleshow/68317790.cms,

be a factor if the particular modality a person needs requires a long drive. For others, anxiety over allowing a stranger to touch them is too high a hurdle. And there's also good old work and school schedules, and childcare concerns. Some people just can't make their schedule line up with the massage therapist's. For all of these reasons, Sacred Massage offers an alternative solution. We *can* get—and give—the loving human touch we need. We just need to learn how.

If you're worried that learning basic massage techniques may be too difficult, remember that we are not aiming to be professionals. There's considerable schooling involved before you can legally call yourself "massage therapist" and charge a fee for your services. However, the bar isn't that high for non-professionals who simply want to work on a loved one, spouse, partner, child, or friend. And we certainly don't need a certificate or license to learn to speak and heal through our touch. We only need a little guidance to get started, to embrace our inner healer, and to offer ourselves as conduits for divine love and compassion. Sprinkle a little magic over all that, and you have Sacred Massage. What may surprise you most is that you already know many of the touch techniques used in massage, but just haven't used them for that purpose. Many of these massage techniques are movements you've already made many, many times—just not in this specific way. As we journey forward, these spiritual and physical skills already within you will rise to the surface and blossom like a lotus arising through murky water.

Touch Heals

Basic massage promotes stress reduction and relaxation, reduces pain, muscle soreness, and tension, improves circulation and immune function, increases energy and alertness, and lowers heart rate and blood pressure. Advanced, specialized massage therapies, called "modalities," have been shown to benefit anxiety, digestive disorders, fibromyalgia, headaches, insomnia, back and neck pain, myofascial pain, nerve pain, soft tissue strains and injuries, sports injuries, and joint pain.[5] Massage therapy can provide relief for arthritis, Alzheimer's disease, autism spectrum disorder, dementia, depression, grief, attention deficit disorder, sensory processing disorder, inflammation, chronic pain, high blood pressure, muscle soreness or cramps, neck and back pain, and swelling after an injury or surgery.[6]

---

5. Mayo Clinic Staff, "Massage: Get in Touch With its Many Benefits," Mayo Clinic, January 12, 2021, https://www.mayoclinic.org/healthy-lifestyle/stress-management/in-depth/massage/art-20045743.

6. Tiffany Field, "Massage Therapy Research Review," National Library of Medicine, April 23, 2016, https://www.ncbi.nlm.nih.gov/pmc/articles/PMC5564319/.

There are also modalities for very specific needs, like easing the effects of chemotherapy, or working on pregnant women, babies, or the frail elderly, as well as modalities to supplement hospice care and ease end-of-life situations. If your loved one is dealing with any of these conditions, it doesn't mean you can't do massage on them it means you'll need to collaborate with their physician to customize your Sacred Massage to best suit your loved one and help them cope with their difficulties and discomforts.

Sacred Massage is a gentle modality and falls in the "basic" category. It aims to provide relaxation, stress reduction, and pain relief that's safe and soothing for most people. If your loved one needs more than that, consult their doctor before proceeding. Don't assume that you *or* your loved one already know what's causing that shoulder pain, and start working out their "knots." That pain might be a torn rotator cuff, and your massage might make it worse. That's the opposite of healing! Conversely, even gentle Sacred Massage might be too much for very fragile people. You need to know what you're dealing with before you start dealing with it.

After an exam, a physician may advise further consultation with a medical specialist, bloodwork, x-rays or a magnetic resonace imaging (MRI), a dietician, lifestyle changes, physical therapy, or even psychotherapy—or a combination thereof. A physician can also advise which massage techniques are safe for your loved one and which should be avoided, and you can tailor your Sacred Massage around that. You can supplement your loved one's professional treatment with massage, and facilitate health and healing, because you have something going for you that all the professionals don't: your love for that person. And they'll feel it in your touch.

Touch Eases Pain

When we think of relieving pain, we usually think of reaching for the bottle of ibuprofen. However, massage can relieve pain, as can simple human touch. According to Michael Changaris, author of *Touch: The Neurobiology of Health, Healing, and Human Connection*, considerable research shows that "simply holding the hand of a person in pain helps reduce their pain-level."[7] A summary of a University of Colorado at Boulder revealed that when a couple holds hands, their heart and breathing rates synchronize, the intensity of pain subsides, and that this "interpersonal synchronization" suggests that a partner's touch has an

---

7. Michael Changaris, *Touch: The Neurobiology of Health, Healing, and Human Connection* (Mendocino, CA: LifeRhythm and Core Evaluation Publications, 2015), 24.

analgesic effect.[8] The lead researcher in this study, Arthur Goldstein, was inspired to study the pain-relieving properties of loving touch while witnessing the birth of his daughter. Seeing his wife in excruciating pain, he wished to help her, and reached for her hand. He saw that his touch helped her, and set out to see if scientific data would corroborate this. The study involved twenty-two established heterosexual couples, and showed that their heart and breathing tended to synchronize simply by sitting next to each other, some holding hands, some not. When the woman was subjected to pain without touching her husband, "that synchronization was severed. When he was allowed to hold her hand, their rates fell into sync again and her pain decreased."

"It could be that touch is a tool for communicating empathy, resulting in an analgesic, or pain-killing, effect," said Goldstein.

While this study involved couples, it's not hard to extrapolate those results to any closely bonded relationship: spouses, partners, parent and child, siblings, or friends. The simple loving, comforting touch of another well-known and trusted person can ease pain, reduce stress, and promote healing.

In another study of couples, sixteen married women were subjected to an electric shock while undergoing a MRI. Some held their husband's hand, some held the hand of an anonymous male experimenter, and some held no hand at all. The brain activity of the women in the first group showed a much lower "threat response" than the women who held a stranger's hand, and that group showed a lower threat response than the women who did not have a hand to hold.[9] In other words, those women who held their spouse's hand experienced less anxiety when anticipating pain, and even a stranger's hand was better than no hand at all.

Why Does It Work?

A National Public Radio story by Michelle Trudeau reveals that when we are touched, it stimulates our "Pacinian corpuscles," which are located in the deep layers of the skin throughout the body and respond to pressure. When stimulated, they in turn stimulate the vagus nerve, which runs from the brain to the abdomen and regulates internal organ func-

8. University of Colorado at Boulder, "When Lovers Touch, Their Breathing, Heartbeat Syncs, Pain Wanes, Study Shows," ScienceDaily, June 21, 2017, https://www.sciencedaily.com/releases/2017/06/170621125313.htm

9. James Q. Coan, Hlllary S. Schaefer, Richard J. Davidson, "Lending a hand: social regulation of the neural response to threat," National Library of Medicine, December 2006, https://pubmed.ncbi.nlm.nih.gov/17201784/.

tions, including digestion, heart rate, and respiratory rate. It is part of the parasympathetic nervous system, which regulates the "flight or fight" response and the body's response to rest and relaxation.[10] According to Trudeau, the vagus nerve responds to gentle, safe pressure with a calming response, including lowering blood pressure and heart rate. Touch from a trusted loved one increases the release of oxytocin, a hormone that promotes trust and bonding. Loving, friendly touch also stimulates the orbital frontal cortex in the brain, which responds to rewarding stimuli like sweets and pleasant scents.[11] This is all just from a simple touch, such as holding a hand, or patting a shoulder. Consider how magnified these neurological and biochemical responses are during a massage, when the Pacinian corpuscles are being stimulated all over the body for an hour. No wonder massage feels so heavenly! In addition to the sensation of our skin and muscles being soothed, our vagus nerve and one of our pleasure centers are also being caressed, bathing our brains in lovely, soothing oxytocin. In other words, massage is more than just skin-deep. It's an entire neurological experience.

At its most basic, massage just makes us feel good. Calm. Serene. Safe. If your loved one doesn't have any particular physical or emotional issue, and all you're really interested in is learning to provide a pleasant, soothing experience, that's reason enough to learn Sacred Massage. However, you'll also be learning techniques to address minor pain, stiffness, and soreness. You'll be able to improve the quality of your loved one's life, no matter what they're struggling with, or even if they're not struggling at all. You already have some pretty impressive healing skills, and you haven't even learned anything yet. Right now, you already have the ability to stimulate someone's Pacinian corpuscles, vagus nerve, and orbital frontal cortex, to lower someone's heart and breathing rates, and to trigger a release of oxytocin. All you have to do is touch them. Wow! How amazing is *that*? Embrace those magnificent healing skills, you healer, you!

Touch Is Life

Humans literally cannot thrive, or survive, without touch. Beginning in infancy, human touch is crucial for survival. Deprived of touch, infants will ultimately fail to thrive, stop

---

10. Physiopedia, "Vagus Nerve," Physiopedia.com, accessed July 16, 2022, https://www.physio-pedia.com/Vagus_Nerve.

11. Michelle Trudeau, "Human Connections Start With A Friendly Touch," National Public Radio, September 20, 2010, https://www.npr.org/templates/story/story.php?storyId=128795325.

eating, and wither and die.[12] Although it sounds brutal, and borderline inhumane, Changaris tells in his book of studies done on children in orphanages (most notoriously, Romanian orphanages, where parentless or abandoned children and babies were essentially warehoused), which reveal that even if all an infant's nutritional and basic physical needs are met, without comforting human touch, the infant won't survive.

"Continual lack of touch and care causes an infant to simply give up," says Changaris, describing how when an infant cries, if no one responds, its behavior will quickly escalate in an attempt to attract help: crying harder and louder, and becoming more and more tense. If its cries go unattended, the infant will become exhausted and the crying will lessen, further reducing the chances that help will arrive. In time, the infant will give up, and stop eating, drinking, or crying, and without intervention, will die.

Wow. Isn't *that* a punch right to the heart.

Changaris notes that an infant needs three basic things in order to survive: security, nourishment, and love—love in the form of loving human touch. The institutionalized infants only received the first two. But that wasn't enough, he concludes.

"To an infant, love communicated by touch, by contact with their caregiver, is as vital as food. Without touch, babies perish."[13]

Although the examples from the orphanages are extreme, it doesn't mean that lack of loving touch isn't detrimental to our physical, psychological, and emotional health. Touch is vital to our health and survival throughout our lives. As children, the adults in our lives (hopefully) meet our physical and emotional needs. As adults, we're able to care for our own security and nourishment, and attend to our own needs and physical discomforts. However, it's really difficult to provide loving touch to ourselves. Hugging and patting ourselves just isn't the same as receiving it from another person. Even if we become very practiced at ignoring and suppressing the need for loving touch and physical comfort, it's always simmering at the edges of our consciousness, yearning for satiation. We just get really good at ignoring it. Well, sort of. We may fill that emotional gap in another way, with an "aholic": workaholic, shopaholic, alcoholic. We circumvent our core need for loving touch with pleasurable and addictive things, that satisfy for the moment, but not in the long run. It works for a day, but the next, we're craving it again, unaware that what we're desperately craving is loving human touch, not a bag of chocolate chip cookies or three more pairs of shoes.

---

12. Changaris, *Touch: The Neurobiology of Health, Healing, and Human Connection*, 18.

13. Changaris, *Touch: The Neurobiology of Health, Healing, and Human Connection*, 18.

This may sound a little backwards, but our problem is that we've become *too* tough. It's much easier to don our psychological armor and brace ourselves against what we really need and want than it is to face and embrace our own vulnerability. For some, it's more difficult to ask for a hug than for another martini. No matter our situation, no matter our age, the basic core need of loving human touch is perpetually yearning to be fulfilled, and it will take what it can get—for the moment. Tomorrow, it's back again, pining for touch.

For those of us lucky enough to have loving friends and family around us, the need for human touch gets satiated, particularly if we have a partner, spouse, or other person to cuddle or be cuddled by. However, access to that life-sustaining touch wanes right along with our years, particularly if that person passes on. Shattered by grief, we continue forth, constantly, deeply, aching for their touch.

Lack of tender human contact is especially pernicious and painful as we advance into our senior years. Elderly people who live in isolation, who have lost a spouse or partner, or are in an assisted or skilled living situation, are often not touched by anyone but nurses or caregivers, who may treat that person as a "thing" that needs to be cleaned up, fed, and medicated, not as a "thou": a living human being in need of a gentle pat on the shoulder or stroke of the cheek, or just simply having a hand held. Becoming a "thing" is arguably more crippling and emotionally devastating than any physical affliction. Right when we need assistance and support more than any time since infancy, we're left to languish and slowly roll to a stop. Oh, what a life-sustaining difference regular loving touch could make in our advanced senior years, when our hunger for life-sustaining touch still burns, but the people and things that give us joy slowly peel away, further amplifying our need for touch. We feel it just as intensely as we did in infancy, but there's no one to satisfy it. Without any loving human touch, our will to live dissolves, and death comes earlier—just like those babies in the Romanian orphanage.

The core need of loving human touch, although amplified at the bookends of our lives, is nonetheless present all that while in between. However, during those middle years, our skin hunger gets muffled by school, jobs, children, family, and all of life's other issues, troubles, and trials. We're so distracted by everything else that recognizing (let alone satisfying) our need for touch gets pushed off our radar. But it's still there, calling out for satiation, even as we're suppressing it and soldiering on anyway.

Most of us manage to find satisfying and meaningful ways to spend our lifetime, even if perpetually craving loving human touch. We try to be good, decent people, and treat others well, find activities to make our lives feel pleasant and worthwhile, and hopefully find employment that is satisfying and pays our bills. We do what we can, and we manage to get by—anyway. But there are those others. I have to wonder about those who don't manage to navigate life successfully under the constant strain of touch starvation. I have to wonder about those who act out their pain with anger and rage, just like an infant whose needs aren't being met, thrashing and shrieking. I have to wonder if the vast array of human tragedies and cruelties—from suicide to homicide, and just plain meanness—could be diminished if everyone received the regular loving touch we all need to live and thrive; if everyone felt safe and loved.

From Motherhood to Massage

Although I learned the techniques of touch in massage school, it was my babies that taught me about the true value of touch. I wasn't a "let them cry" mom. I took my mothering cues from animals, not my own background. Mama cats don't let their kittens cry. They go to them immediately, and soothe them. If my babies cried, I picked them up and held them close. I sang to them and rocked them to sleep every night, well into toddlerhood. And the comfort went both ways. The feeling of a limp, warm, relaxed, squishy baby against your chest—that's some powerful medicine for chronic skin hunger.

Rocking my babies to sleep and gazing upon their sweet, peaceful faces provided the epiphany for drawing the line between love and massage, from which my spiritual, magical approach to massage grew. A couple years into my massage practice, I was finishing up a massage as always: seated behind the end of the massage table, cradling the client's head in my hands, just resting in that quiet moment. I gazed down at her face and for the first time, really *noticed* it: completely relaxed, completely peaceful. Just like my babies. That triggered a motherly rush of warm love and compassion for this person, and right then, it hit me: Massage isn't just about loosening tight muscles and relieving aches and pains, or even about relaxation per se. It's much more than that. It's about creating a safe cocoon that allows people to sink into a deep state of childlike bliss and pure trust. Just like my babies, my clients feel so safe under my hands that their stress and worries just melt away. Massage can bring out the "sleeping infant" in most anyone, and how loving and special that is—to trust someone so deeply and completely that they'll allow you to hold their entire existence in your hands. Massage isn't a service. It's a relationship. A trusting, compassionate, *sacred* relationship.

That was the moment when my approach to massage changed. In addition to pain relief and relaxation, every session became an opportunity to invite and channel divine love, caring, compassion, and healing into our time together. Every session could be magical. Every session could be sacred.

Activity
MEDITATION FOR EMBRACING LOVE AND COMPASSION

This meditation guides you to open up to love and compassion, and learn to direct it. You must have love and compassion within you, for yourself, before you can transmit them to someone else. You must connect to your own inner peace in order to channel peace through your touch.

To do this meditation, find a time and place where you won't be disturbed for about fifteen minutes. Read through the steps a couple times and memorize them. To help you memorize these steps, rather than attempting to meditate and visualize while reading from a book (which is utterly impossible), assign each step to a finger. Touch your fingertip to your thumb for each step as a prompt to help you remember them. Before beginning, make yourself comfortable (seated or lying down) and get a blanket or pillow if you wish. Turn off your phone and devices.

Breathe and clear (index finger). Close your eyes, and just breathe. Focus on your breath flowing in, and flowing back out, without any effort. Just breathe comfortably and naturally. Quiet your thoughts. If a thought interrupts, simply acknowledge it—*Oh, that's a thought*—and mentally just swipe it away. Return to your internal quiet space, and keep breathing. Note the safe, firm surface supporting you. Gravity pulls on your body—that's Mother Earth pulling you close. Let her hold you. Tell yourself, *"I am safe."*

Visualize (middle finger). Visualize your arms folded together at your chest, cradling a sweet, innocent, sleeping baby. Relax into the image and gaze at its long eyelashes and delicate hair, chubby cheeks, and little rosebud mouth. Feel the weight of that baby in your arms and against your chest, completely relaxed, completely peaceful, breathing softly and regularly. Open your heart and pour love onto that child. Feel the love flowing. Open yourself up to Spirit, and invite divine love from the universe to pour into you…through you…enveloping that baby. Relax in this moment of free-flowing love and compassion. Feel its richness and immensity. Feel your heart warm and swell. Stay in this moment for as long as you like.

Turn your love inward (ring finger). Focus on the love and compassion you feel for that sweet baby, grab ahold of it, and curl it back onto yourself. Divert that warm feeling directly into you. Let it well up. Allow yourself to feel and receive all the love you felt for that baby for just yourself. Let it flow through you, into you, wrap around you like a soft blanket. Relax into this experience, and let that self-love swell and swirl. Softly whisper or think, "I love you so much." Bask in this saturation of infinite love and compassion for as long as you like.

Refocus on breathing (pinky). With divine love swirling within you, return your attention to your breathing. Focus on your breath flowing in effortlessly, and flowing back out, comfortably and naturally. Quiet your thoughts. If a thought interrupts, acknowledge it, and mentally swipe it away. Notice the safe, firm surface supporting you. Notice Mother Earth, still pulling you close. Tell yourself, *"I am safe."* When you feel ready, open your eyes and return to the room where you began your meditation. Carry that divine love and compassion within you as you continue through your day.

Return to this meditation any time you feel tender or raw, or whenever life seems harsh or unhelpful. You can do this meditation anytime, anywhere, and if anyone around you questions you, just say you're resting your eyes. Which you are…along with your spirit. You don't even need a reason. You can do it "just because." This is a perfect meditation to practice just before falling asleep—wrap yourself in a warm blanket of divine love and compassion, and complete safety.

Opening up to divine love and compassion, receiving it, and directing it to flow through you toward someone else makes you a more intuitive and effective healer. However, just filling yourself with these feelings is self-nourishing and healing. That has value! As the old saying goes, "You can't pour from an empty cup." Keep your own cup of divine love full to the brim.

Activity
Meditation for Directing Love and Compassion

Now that you've experienced directing infinite, divine love and compassion toward yourself, you'll learn to continue directing it through you and toward someone else. Repeat the exact same meditation, but after infusing yourself with nurturing love, imagine streaming it from your heart, down through your arms, and right into the palms of your hands. Feel your hands holding all that love and compassion. They may start to feel warm, and even tingly.

We already know that plain old touch can heal. Imagine how that healing power increases exponentially when your touch is infused with divine love and compassion channeled straight from Spirit, through your own heart, and right out of your hands.

They Can Feel What You Think

In addition to healing, love, and compassion, there's something else that can be transmitted through touch: energy and images generated by your thoughts and feelings. If you're having painful thoughts or feelings, or are distracted by worries or plans, your loved one may sense that something isn't quite right. They may not be able to identify specifically what that something is, but they'll feel your unsettled energy. If your energy feels "off," your loved one's experience will also feel "off." Difficult thoughts and feelings will seep right into your touch, and your loved one will notice, making it more difficult for them to relax. They will feel distracted, because *you* are distracted. Distraction is not helpful for massage—not for you, and not for your loved one.

If your distracted thoughts are about cuddly kittens or chocolate cream pie, that probably won't create frenetic or upsetting energy. However, if the tragedy-du-jour on the evening news is tumbling through your mind like shoes in the dryer, it will be conveyed in your touch. One of the main reasons to "ground and center" (which we'll discuss in depth later on) is to clear your mind of distracting or upsetting worries, thoughts, or feelings, *before* starting your massage session. Rather than focusing on your problems, you turn your focus toward your own breathing, your own body, the ground beneath your feet, and then your loved one. Even then, distracting thoughts can sometimes break through your defenses.

We learned about how thoughts can be transmitted through touch in massage school. We sat face to face with a partner, our eyes closed, holding hands. One person was the "giver," and visualized something of our choice, viewing it from every angle, and imagining the touch, taste, sound, or feel of that thing in as much detail as possible. The "receiver" simply cleared their mind and opened it to any images that came floating through.

In this exercise, I was the giver. I envisioned a huge puff of sweet pink fluffy cotton candy. We sat holding hands for awhile, visualizing and receiving. We were then told to open our eyes, and one by one, the receivers revealed the images they saw. Just as I was thinking, "Yeah, right—this is dumb," my partner described the "pink fluffy clouds" he saw. Good thing I was sitting on the floor, or I would've fallen out of my chair. It wasn't "precisely" cotton candy, but it was close enough. He'd gotten the gist of it. As we went around the circle, in almost every pair, the image received was too close to the giver's thoughts to be random. I remember another pair, where the giver thought of a barber's pole, and the receiver envisioned candy canes. That's much too similar to be a lucky guess.

We learned that day that whatever fills your mind can infiltrate your touch, and negatively affect your massage session. Just because thoughts and feelings are between your ears doesn't mean they won't filter out through your hands. I got a real-life reminder of this lesson years later, while beginning a massage with a client that knew me well and was particularly intuitive. I'd gotten really rattled over something just before her appointment, and I don't even remember what the issue was, only that I was all wrapped around the axle about it. I attempted to shelve that issue for the time being, cleared my head, and went into the room to start my session, but the issue kept poking my mind in the ribs. I grounded, I centered, and was clear and focused on our session—or so I thought. However, the moment I placed my hands on her, she said, "What's wrong? Your energy is off."

There's no pretending in Sacred Massage, and there was no point denying it because she already felt my "off" energy. You can't un-ring that bell. So, I briefly acknowledged it and told her not to worry about it, but she insisted that we talk it out right there and then. Now, talking about your own issues during a massage is a full stop "no." That hour belongs to my client, not me. But this person had already detected my poorly suppressed funky energy, and there's no disingenuity in Sacred Massage either. Like the old saying goes, "Don't piss on my shoes and tell me it's raining." So, I broke my rule about discussing personal issues, aired my grievances, and then we were able to proceed as normal.

Just remember: if you think it, they can feel it.

Activity
PRACTICING THOUGHTFUL TOUCH

You can experiment with how thoughts can affect your touch by trying it on yourself. Without making any effort to alter your thoughts or feelings, place your palm on top of your arm or thigh, and run it up and back. Note how that feels. Probably okay, right? No problem.

Now, close your eyes, and think or say to yourself, "Everything is fine. I am safe. I am loved." Continue thinking or saying that as you run your palm up and back down again. Did it feel different? Did the quality of your touch change? Was your experience of that touch different?

Try this with a friend or partner. Without telling them what you're doing, touch them without clearing your mind—hold their hand or run your hand up and down their arm. Next, focus your mind on something you absolutely love, like cookies baking in the oven or floating in a pool, and repeat the touch. Ask them if there was a difference. You could even try that massage school "giver and receiver" imagery exercise and see what happens. You may be amazed!

Many Types of Touch

We've been talking about touch and massage in a very generalized way so far. However, the language of touch has many dialects, or "modalities." Regardless of the type of touch, their origins are simple, soothing human contact. While we can't document the very first human touch, we can track the history of massage, which stretches back centuries, with documented practices in India, Egypt, Greece, Rome, Sweden, China, Japan, and many more, with each culture offering many different techniques and practices. Massage practices across cultures and through time were often associated with health and healing, and some were even considered to be medical treatment. Modern massage borrows heavily from these cross-cultural origins, such as the slow, sweeping movements of Swedish massage, and "Acupressure" or "Trigger Point Therapy," with their roots in Chinese medicine, and Shiatsu, which developed in Japan.

Massage appeared in the United States as early as the 1700s, when "rubbers" worked with doctors to treat various conditions with rubbing and friction.[14] Today, there is a cornucopia of massage modalities available, and strictly in the interest of research (*wink, wink*), it's optimal to experience as many modalities as you can. It'll be the most pleasant course of study ever! Besides learning about different modalities, just learning to receive touch and relax into another person's hands will enhance and accelerate your skills when providing massage for a friend or loved one. When you fall in love with being touched and the experience of being saturated in serenity, you'll naturally want to share that experience with someone else.

Following are some brief descriptions of a few common massage modalities. Pick some that interest you and make an appointment with a massage therapist that practices

---

14. Florida Academy, "The History of Massage Therapy: 5,000 Years of Relaxation and Pain Relief," May 17, 2019, https://florida-academy.edu/history-of-massage-therapy/.

that modality. Find out what you like and don't like, and you might also pick up a technique or two that you want to try yourself. These modalities may differ by philosophy, approach, method, and style, or may address specific needs, such as age or health condition, and it's not an exhaustive list. There are many, many more massage modalities, and even veterinary modalities for horses, cats, and dogs. Whatever the condition, age, or even species, there's a modality to suit that need.

Acupressure

Acupressure is pressure applied with the thumbs or fingers into specific points on the body to relieve muscular tension and increase blood circulation. It's believed to activate our life force (also called qi or chi), which promotes healing. These points are also used by acupuncturists, who use fine needles to stimulate these points. Acupuncture and acupressure activate the energy meridians in the body, and some therapists may incorporate Chinese herbal medicine into their practice. Both practices have their roots in ancient Chinese healing practices in which certain areas are stimulated with pressure or needles to relieve pain not only at that spot, but also to transfer relief to other areas of the body as well, including organs, which are believed to be stimulated by those specific points.

Aromatherapy

Essential oils can enhance the mood and tone of a massage experience, and most oils have a specific purpose, such as relaxation, stimulation, or improving circulation. The oils are extracted from herbs, flowers, roots, woods, and resins. The oils are usually blended into a neutral carrier oil. The oils may be dissipated into a room via a diffuser and some are applied directly to the skin full strength or blended into massage oil or lotion.

Ayurveda

The practice of Ayurveda stretches back 5,000 years in India, where it is considered a medical treatment. Ayurvedic practices stretch beyond the massage table, and encompass diet, detoxification, and lifestyle choices. Ayurvedic massage is a full-body detoxification treatment, using warmed oil, particularly sesame oil. Ayurveda considers the impact and needs of three basic body/constitution types called doshas: vata, pitta, and kapha. Ayurveda also encompasses an understanding of the five elements (ether, air, fire, water, and earth).

Chair Massage

Chair massage is done just like how it sounds: in a chair, and usually fully clothed. There are special massage chairs for this modality, and it's a common service at airports, shopping malls, street fairs, marathons, or competitive sporting events where it's inconvenient or impractical to disrobe. It's useful for someone who can't get onto a massage table, or doesn't feel comfortable disrobing, or both.

Deep Tissue

Deep tissue massage presses deeper than the skin and surface muscles, down into the inside layers as well as the attachments of the muscles and tendons, and the connective tissue known as "fascia." It can be very intense. Deep tissue techniques release tension and increase range of motion in the deepest layers of muscle tissue, tendons and fascia. It can alleviate chronic muscle pain and tightness, and reduce inflammation. This modality is often incorporated into sports massage, which aims to relieve pain and increase mobility particularly for people who regularly participate in sports or other physically demanding activities.

Geriatric Massage

This modality is light and gentle, and specifically tailored for the elderly, but is also appropriate for anyone who is physically fragile. Knowledge about the aging process is part of the training for geriatric massage, and extra care is given to thin, delicate skin, stiff joints, and brittle bones. Some who specialize in geriatric massage practice in retirement homes and residential care facilities. This modality can improve the well-being of those who are not physically active or must stay in a wheelchair or even in bed. Geriatric massage can also relieve stress and anxiety, and improve sleep.

Healing Touch

Although "healing touch" is a general term you'll often hear in massage discussions, when capitalized, it refers to a specific modality. Light touch (and sometimes no touch at all) manipulates the energy fields in the body, and promotes physical and emotional healing and relaxation. This modality can be done fully clothed. Like Reiki, the focus is more on the energy field surrounding the body than on touching the body. Healing Touch is quiet, calming, and gentle, and should be tolerated by even the most fragile or sensitive individuals.

Hot Stone

Smooth, heated stones are fantastic for warming up the body and facilitating relaxation before doing massage. Stones of varying sizes are heated in very warm water, and then placed along the back and even between the toes to warm the body. Large, smooth, warmed stones are then used to spread oil slowly and firmly into sore, tight muscles. This slow, smooth, warming modality is deeply relaxing. Cold stones are also sometimes used on particular spots, such as tight spots in the neck or wherever inflammation may be a factor.

Infant Massage

Just like geriatric massage is tailored to an elderly person's needs, this modality is tailored to another fragile type of person: infants. New parents can learn infant massage to improve the bonding process and relax a fussy or cranky baby. Nothing upsets a parent more than a squalling infant that will not be calmed. This modality can coax an infant to relax and even fall asleep. It may also relieve colic. Infant Massage may be helpful for premature infants and even practiced in the hospital while the infant is still in the neonatal care unit.

Lymphatic Drainage

This modality requires a very light touch, like butterfly wings, which helps move lymph from swollen areas, such as hands and feet. There are lymph nodes all over the body, and to help lymph drain, the nodes between the swollen area and the heart are first gently pumped with flat fingers, followed by light brushing from the swollen area to a nearby node in the direction of the heart. This modality can be beneficial for relieving edema (swelling) from illness, injury, surgery, or chemotherapy.

Myofascial Release

The fascia (connective tissue) in our bodies can become tight and inflamed, just like our muscles. Fascia covers our organs, bones, muscles, tendons, and ligaments. When it's healthy, it's slippery and smooth. When it's not, it becomes thick, sticky, and tight. This modality uses gentle pressure to release restrictions in the fascia, as well as stimulation of trigger points.

Oncology Massage

People living with cancer or undergoing treatment must endure considerable discomfort from radiation, chemotherapy, surgery, and the disease process itself. This modality is specialized to offer cancer patients relief from the discomfort and anxiety they're experiencing, in all stages of the disease, from treatment to recovery to survivor to terminal.

Prenatal/Pregnancy Massage

Although pregnancy is an amazing phase of life for most women, discomfort is part of the gig. In the early months, there's morning sickness. As the fetus grows, mothers may experience swelling in the legs and feet, backaches, and navigating their rapidly changing body shape and weight. Pregnancy massage is often offered in a side-lying position because it's safer for both mother and fetus this way. There are also body cushions especially made for pregnant women to allow them to feel more comfortable and relaxed on the table. Prenatal massage helps a woman relax, and may ease anxiety and pain during labor.

Reflexology

The theory behind reflexology is that certain points or zone on the body correspond to various organs and areas of the body. Stimulating these points and zones (in a fashion similar to acupressure) can relieve a variety of issues and discomfort in their corresponding body parts. Feet and hands in particular have complex and detailed points and zones for providing relief, improving circulation, and reducing pain and stress. This modality is helpful for someone who can't tolerate a lot of skin contact or friction, such as a burn victim, someone recovering from injuries or surgery that require them to remain still or lying down, someone weakened from advanced disease, or with very sensitive fibromyalgia.

Reiki

Reiki healing is all about energy. Originating in Japan, Reiki heals through the connection to the sacred life force (chi) and channeling it to another person. Sometimes the therapist will place hands lightly on the client's body, and sometimes the hands will not touch at all, but will remain within that person's energy field. Reiki is even practiced from a distance, with therapist and client possibly not in the same room, town, or state. A certified Reiki therapist has received the sacred Reiki symbols directly from a Reiki master. The symbols are passed directly from master to student, over the generations, in a continuous line. These sessions are still, quiet, and calming, and excellent for emotional stress or anxiety, and often done fully clothed.

Sacred Massage

Well, of *course* we're going to include Sacred Massage on this list! Sacred Massage incorporates Soothing Touch massage techniques into an overall spiritual, magical experience. It's like going to a concert. The overall event is the Sacred Massage, from the time you enter the concert hall to the time you leave. The physical playing of music on the instruments is the Soothing Touch. A memorable, satisfying concert requires both—the music *and* the atmosphere. Sacred Massage is intended for non-professionals to provide relaxation and relief to friends and loved ones. Sacred Massage elevates a basic relaxation massage to a spiritual experience, conducted as a magical ritual.

Shiatsu

Like Reiki, Shiatsu originated in Japan, and employs delivering pressure with thumb, fingers, palms, elbows, and even knees to particular points and energy meridians on the body, which correspond to certain other areas or spots in the body. They are the same points and zones used in acupuncture and acupressure. This applied pressure (which can be very intense) assists these spots in releasing, and encourages healing in the corresponding areas and throughout the body.

Sports Massage

Sports massage aims to improve and enhance athletic performance and recovery before, during, or after a workout, event, or competition. It is also used to treat and prevent sports-related injury. This modality is at the deep end of the pressure spectrum and can be very intense. It often parallels techniques used in physical therapy, and may focus on a particular area or issue, rather than a full-body treatment. Sports massage is often offered on-site at sporting events and competitions, and can sometimes be done fully clothed.

Swedish Massage

Swedish massage is possibly the most familiar modality, and often the starting point for many massage therapists' careers. The slow, sweeping, relaxing Swedish strokes over the soft tissues of the body are accompanied by kneading and pressing. Swedish massage is a go-to modality for simple relaxation and improved circulation. This modality is commonly offered in spas and massage offices.

Thai

Thai massage comes from—surprise—Thailand. The origins of this modality can be traced back more than 2,000 years to India, and credited to Shivago Komarpaj, the personal physician of the Buddha. Thai massage is done on a firm mat on the floor rather than on a massage table, with the client fully clothed. The therapist uses leverage and pressure from their own body weight to release tension and improve circulation. Like Shiatsu and Reflexology, Thai massage creates internal effects in the body by stimulating certain external points on the body.

Trigger Point

Like Shiatsu, Reflexology, and Myofascial Release, Trigger Point Therapy involves focused compression or pressing, massaging, and stretching particular spots to relieve pain and stiffness. It has much in common with Myofascial Release, and is also used to get the fascia moving smoothly and easily again. Other benefits include increased range of motion, pain reduction, and improved function. Trigger points are particular spots or tight "knots" in the body, and can occur in a variety of places.

This is but a tiny sample of the many massage modalities available. For an expanded list of modalities, visit the Associated Bodywork & Massage Professionals (ABMP)[15] website. The ABMP is a good resource for finding more information about specific modalities, and for finding a practitioner of those modalities near you.

Becoming a Healer

We've barely scratched the (skin!) surface of all the massage modalities available, and new modalities are being developed all the time. There are even modalities that make use of seashells or colored light. Their common denominator is that all (with the exception of Sacred Massage) involve a trained professional manipulating bodily tissue or energy fields

---

15. Associated Bodywork & Massage Professionals (ABMP), "Find a Massage Therapist or Bodyworker," accessed November 5, 2021, https://www.massagetherapy.com/glossary.

to produce a feeling of relief or relaxation, and to promote healing. Some modalities use tools, some don't.

I've borrowed from many of these modalities to develop my massage techniques and sequences, some of which I'll share with you. These physical techniques will be known collectively as Soothing Touch, the "working" section of a Sacred Massage experience. The spiritual, magical components complete the session as Sacred Massage, and you'll learn those techniques as well.

This journey won't be about striving to become a massage therapist, but rather, for you to connect with your inner healer; to learn how to channel compassion, love, healing, and divine energy through touch; and to incorporate magical concepts and practices to elevate a regular massage into a healing ritual. Our Sacred Massage journey is all about accessing the comfort, compassion, and healing abilities already within you that are ready to blossom. You'll learn to truly embrace your new title—not massage therapist, but "healer."

Chapter 2

What You'll Need

Before we pull the massage sheet back and start learning the steps and sequences of doing massage, there are a few things you're going to need because optimally, they will make your massage session go more smoothly and comfortably for both you and your loved one. However, budgets and situations aren't always optimal. In these cases, we must get innovative and figure out how to make it work. If you can't afford all these items, don't despair. You can improvise and find creative alternatives or substitutions. And remember, you could do an entire Sacred Massage session without any tools at all except your love, compassion, a little divinity, a little magic, and those healing hands. Things are great, but *you* are really the only component that makes Sacred Massage happen.

Massage Table

A massage table is first on this list because it is literally the platform for learning the massage sequences, as well as doing massage on your loved one. In addition, you'll learn in the section on magic that it serves a dual purpose for transforming your massage into a magical practice—it becomes a magical altar. If you invest in only one thing for doing massage, let it be a massage table. It doesn't have to be an expensive, professional-grade table—it can be used, or a freebie hand-me-down. You can buy a new table on a massage supply website (massagewarehouse.com is my go-to), but you don't have to whack your wallet to find one. They're often available at discount warehouse stores for a fraction of the cost, and easily found on Craigslist or social media pages dedicated to local sales or certain types of items. You can also acquire a table (or pretty much anything) with a simple social media post: "Hey, friends! I need a massage table." You may even get more responses than you anticipated. Make it known in your community and on your social media pages that you need a used table, or need to borrow one. Announce this need wherever, and to whomever, you can think of. The universe can't connect you with what you want unless you let it know what you're looking for!

I recommend a portable table, which can be left up all the time, if you like, or folded up and stored behind a door. You can also take it with you if your loved one can't come to your home, and most come with a carrying case. Although the tables look big, most are under forty pounds, and the carrying cases have a cross-body shoulder strap that makes them pretty easy to move around. There are also massage table carts if you don't want to carry the table.

If a table just isn't possible right now, that's okay. Don't let the lack of a table thwart you. Be open to the possibility that the universe will direct a table to you—if you ask. You may not have a table right at the moment—but you will. In the meantime, you can improvise.

Massaging without a Table

If getting a massage table seems like an insurmountable obstacle, compensate by using what is available to you. You can work on a bed, but it will be hard on your body because you'll have to do a lot of stooping and bending over, as the surface is too low to stand and work. Leaning over a person's body in an awkward position puts strain on your back and neck. If you don't have any choice but to work on a bed, position your loved one about one body width away from the edge of the bed, and sit down next to them, massaging from this position. To work on the other side of the body, they can either turn around 180 degrees, or move to the other side of the bed.

If you must work on a couch, or the floor, use cushions or folded blankets to create a soft but firm surface that supports the entire length of the body. One option is to remove the cushions from your sofa and line them up on the floor. But again, like working from a bed, the couch or the floor will be a lot harder on you than your loved one. You'll likely have to kneel by the couch, which will be brutal on your knees. You can also work on the floor, but again, you'll have to kneel, and while your loved one may be perfectly comfortable, your knees will hate you.

An important consideration for positioning your loved one facedown without a massage table—whether on a bed, couch, or the floor—is finding a way to prop the head so the neck remains straight, while also allowing enough air flow so your loved one can breathe. Fold or roll some towels or a blanket into a U-shape, and place it at one end of the cushions you lined up to serve as a face cradle, and you could get by with that.

If your loved one is unable to lie on a table, or must remain in a sitting position, there are also massage chairs to do seated massage, and they're easily transported if you must work away from home. If your loved one must remain in a regular chair or wheelchair, or in a hospital bed (or prefers to), you can adapt to these situations too. We'll cover how to adapt for these alternate situations in the last chapter after we learn the complete Sacred Massage sequence, so you'll have a fuller understanding of what you can adapt and what you can't, and how to work around obstacles and challenges.

Whenever the situation is less than optimal, improvise. When you meet an obstacle, don't just sit down and say "Well, that's that." Figure out how to go over it, under it, around it, or through it. (That's also a little freebie life lesson I tossed in there!)

Even if you know you won't ultimately be working on a massage table, you'll still have a better learning experience if you get a table while we learn the Soothing Touch massage techniques and sequences because they are explained with the assumption that your practice partner or loved one is situated on a massage table. A table will make it much easier to comprehend what we're doing, and to practice and learn.

Music

Music really enhances a massage experience. Sweet, ambient instrumental music is most compatible with relaxation. Avoid music with a beat, and music with lyrics. Your brain is hard-wired to attend to words, even if they're in a song. This creates a distraction for your loved one, and we want to minimize distraction. Google "massage music" or "Reiki music," and you'll find a cornucopia of options. My go-to massage musicians are Anugama, Dean Evenson, and Deuter, if you want a place to start. Also, a soundtrack of nothing but ocean waves always works.

If you'll be playing music, CDs will work, but they don't last long for massage. Oil gets on them, which attracts dust and dirt, making them skip. Once they start to skip, they must go in the trash. A skipping track disrupts relaxation. Another downfall for using CDs is that they are usually too short to last a full hour. I have transitioned to using streaming services exclusively, because there's no interruption in the music. Nothing is as loud as sudden silence during a massage. There are several streaming sources with extensive music catalogues and volumes of massage-appropriate music.

Because you'll be playing the music at very low volumes, the quality of the speaker is less important. Couple your phone or tablet with a Bluetooth speaker and that will work just fine. No need for a fancy sound system. Using a device with a speaker is also great for working away from home. If you don't have a speaker, here's a little sound system hack: Put your phone speaker-side down in a coffee cup or pointed toward a wall—the sound will be less tinny. Put your device on "Do Not Disturb" during your session so calls and texts don't come through. The sound of a phone call or text interrupts relaxation, and actually answering the call or text during a massage session is just heinous. It's like telling your loved one that they aren't the most important thing to you at that moment—the polar opposite of a Sacred Massage experience. Whatever it is, it can go to voicemail.

Lighting

Lighting during a massage is crucial. Too bright, and the atmosphere feels harsh. Too low—well, that's almost not a thing. You could do an entire massage by candlelight. The lighting should feel like dusk—neither light nor dark; that sleepy soothing feeling that arises when the sun slips below the violet horizon, and flowers close their petals and birds return to their nests. Dusk means it's time to slow down and rest—and so does massage. Low light and darkness stimulate the pineal gland in the brain, which releases melatonin and induces drowsiness. Bright light does the opposite. If you stare into a phone, computer, or tablet just before bedtime, it's like shining a spotlight into your pineal gland, which interferes with the release of melatonin, which in turn interferes with sleep.

If your massage space has harsh lighting, turn it off and use a small lamp instead. A string of white Christmas lights will also create just enough light for massage, and adds gentle ambiance. Keep lighting to only the bare minimum you need to see what you're doing. Your loved one doesn't need any light at all, and the less, the better.

Sheets and Blankets

Sheets and blankets are an absolute necessity, unless your loved one will remain clothed. You can get sheets made specifically for a massage table, but any set of twin sheets will do. There are face cradle covers, but you can fold a pillowcase to cover the face cradle. Flannel is the gold standard for massage, and feels cozy and comfortable on the skin, but other fabrics will work too. If using cotton sheets, make sure the thread count isn't so low that they're scratchy on bare skin. Professional massage table sheet sets are available online and will fit your table perfectly. Another advantage to professional sheets is that they're thicker and higher quality than most ordinary flannel sheets, and meant for professional wear and tear, as well as many trips through the washing machine.

As for blankets, a throw-sized TV blanket works great. They're a bit larger than a beach towel and often made of fleece, which is warm and comfy. They're also inexpensive and easy to wash. They will probably get oil dribbled on them, so use blankets that you don't mind getting dirty or stained, and can take multiple washings.

When choosing your sheets and blankets, remember your color magic! Pick soothing colors that inspire relaxation, not red-and-yellow plaid or wild purple-and-orange polka dots. Keep it simple, keep it soft. Plain solid pastels or deep earthy colors like dark blue or brown always work.

Table and Face Cradle Covers

Massage oil and lotion will seep through sheets and damage a table and face cradle over time, so they should have protective covers underneath the massage sheet. It can be as simple as a beach towel for the table and hand towel for the cradle, or you can find covers online. The ones made of fleece are wonderful because they add extra softness and warmth. An unpadded face cradle can start to feel hard and uncomfortable on the forehead and cheekbones, so extra padding there is a thoughtful touch. An actual massage table cover also has elastic loops at the corners to keep it in place while you work, rather than sliding around and creating uncomfortable wrinkles and bumps.

If you're not working on a table—a bed, for example—you'll still need to put something protective down before working or the bed sheets and mattress will get greasy. An extra-large beach towel works great because it will catch the oil rather than let it seep through.

Towels

Towels are multi-purpose in massage. Besides just wiping or blotting things, they become makeshift bolsters for elevating or supporting various body parts, allowing your loved one to relax comfortably. A rolled bath towel becomes a bolster under the knees when your loved one is lying on their back, easing strain on the lower back. Facedown, it can be placed just below the collarbone to ease pressure on the breasts. A folded hand towel can lift a small area, such as the shoulder, to alleviate pressure on a joint, injury, or while recovering from surgery. A hand towel can be rolled longwise and placed under the neck while your loved one is on their back, easing pressure on the cervical spine. There are actual massage bolsters for all these purposes, but you can get by just fine with towels. And they're inexpensive and easy to wash.

Pillows

Pillows work when more elevation is needed than a rolled-up towel can provide. Some people need or prefer more leg elevation while on their backs, while others may need to keep their upper body elevated slightly, such as someone with severe acid reflux. Pillows are also necessary for massaging in a side-lying position, such as during pregnancy or after abdominal surgery. Be aware that the pillows may get greasy, so dedicate certain pillows for massage only. They don't have to be expensive, just fluffy. Always cover them with pillowcases to keep them as clean as possible. If they start to smell funky or look stained, and can't be cleaned, they're done. Donate them to a local animal shelter or veterinary office. (And that goes for your massage sheets too.)

Massage Holster and Bottle

These are often sold in sets, usually for less than ten bucks, and they're worth every penny. Having your oil right there and easily accessed lets you do your session without disrupting the flow and contact of your hands. In school, we learned to keep at least one hand on a client's body at all times whenever possible, because in a deeply relaxed state, the sudden cessation of contact disrupts relaxation, just like when music suddenly stops. With a holster and pump bottle strapped around your waist, you can replenish your oil or lotion with one hand, without losing contact with your loved one. Massage holsters and bottles are also great for working away from home.

Massage Oil or Lotion

Massage oil or lotion is necessary for working on bare skin. You want an oil that's thickish, allowing your hands to slide easily (called "glide" in the biz), but also has a little "drag," which means it has enough viscosity to provide the slightest friction, allowing you to control your hands when applying pressure so they don't accidentally shoot off into places they shouldn't. Besides oil or lotion, there are also massage creams, butters, and gels. Whichever you pick is a matter of preference—however, lotion is absorbed by the skin much more quickly than oil, so you'll go through it much faster.

Be very careful about buying "massage oil" anywhere other than a professional massage outlet. Non-professional massage oils can have all sorts of ingredients and chemicals that aren't good for the skin, and many of them are intended for *bom-chicka-mow-mow* massage, not what we're doing here. Sometimes "massage oil" is a *wink-wink* way of saying "lube." Non-professional massage oil also often has entirely too much fragrance, and it's usually a synthetic fragrance, not a natural one. I had a client who convinced me to use her own chocolate-scented massage oil, which she loved. About 30 minutes in, I was nauseous from the overwhelming scent. (Yes, too much chocolate can be a thing.) Another client asked me to use her expensive Estee Lauder "massage lotion" for a special birthday massage. It was so saturated in chemical perfume, I started coughing, sneezing, and wheezing within moments, and felt like my throat was closing up. So, I no longer will work with someone else's oil or lotion unless it's specifically intended for massage or a pure kitchen oil, like olive or sesame. Like lighting, scent should be kept to a pure, bare minimum. If you want scent, stick to essential oils or herbs, not human-made perfume.

When choosing an oil, lotion, or cream for massage, consider that skin isn't merely a covering. It's an actual organ, and will absorb chemicals and substances that can enter the bloodstream. Non-professional lotions and oils can include all sorts of toxic ingredients, like BHA and BHT, parabens, petroleum byproducts, and phthalates.[16] Rubbing toxic ingredients into someone's skin is contrary to healing intentions. Also, "all natural" or "fragrance free" doesn't mean that product is free of chemicals. You must read labels. If the ingredients are mostly long words you can't pronounce—keep looking. Also, be wary of "organic" on a label, unless the product has an official USDA organic seal.

In general, professional massage oils and lotions are safer than commercial ones, because they don't offer products that cause skin irritations or worse. Most professional products are free of harmful chemicals. *Most.* Read the ingredients list anyway. Massage suppliers also offer pure oils, like jojoba or coconut. Some oil blends are scented by their natural ingredients, such as lavender or shea butter, and others are unscented.

Your local grocery store is also a great massage supply outlet. My motto for oils or lotions is "If you can't eat it, don't put it on your skin." If you can use it in the kitchen, you can probably use it for massage too. However, not all oils are created equal. Sure, vegetable oil is edible and will work, but it's kinda gross and may contain genetically modified and non-organic substances. There are better choices, like virgin olive oil, or avocado, coconut, or sesame oils. Always pick an organic oil, so you aren't rubbing pesticide into your loved one's skin.

Sesame oil is a staple in Ayurveda massage, and is a wonderful all-around massage oil. However, toasted sesame oil has a very strong scent. Choose the light-colored oil over

---

16. Honey Girl Organics, "15 Toxic Ingredients in Skin Care and Cosmetics Products," HoneyGirlOrganics, accessed March 22, 2022, https://honeygirlorganics.com/pages/15-toxic-ingredients-in-skin-care.

the dark. I personally love virgin olive oil, but some people find the scent overpowering. Choose a "light" olive oil if the scent is too pungent. Coconut "oil" is a solid at room temperature and melts quickly at 78 degrees—right under your hands as you spread it on. The heavenly scent takes you to a tropical summer oasis. Avocado oil is perfect for just about everything—in the massage room and out. It has almost no scent, but does have a light buttery flavor. You can use it for massage and drizzled over your popcorn.

Sesame, olive, coconut, and avocado oils are more than simply harmless on the skin—they're actually extremely beneficial, particularly for dry skin. Using one of these oils gives you confidence about what you're rubbing into your loved one's skin. Rub any leftover on your hands through the hair, and your loved one can get a mini-hair conditioning treatment bonus. The downside of cooking oils is that they're relatively thick and heavy compared to professional massage oil, and can be more difficult to get out of sheets. They may leave oil stains on your sheets, and your clothes too. (Don't do a massage in any clothing that can't get oil on it.)

As for professional lotions, creams, butters, and gels, there's a myriad of products available. You can also make your own lotions, creams, and herbal oils at home, and be confident about what's in them. Making your own lotion or oil has added magical bonus—you can infuse them with magical intent as you prepare them.

Chair

A chair is for you, not your loved one. When doing much of the upper body work while your loved one is lying faceup, you'll need to sit at the end of the massage table, behind their head. Standing and leaning over, or kneeling, will eventually cause you substantial discomfort. Also, if you're in pain while working on someone else, it negatively affects your touch. There are special massage stools, which have a round seat and roll around easily, but I find a padded folding chair works just great. It's much cheaper and can be stored behind a door.

Clock

If you need to keep track of time, any clock will do as long as you can see the hands and numbers easily. A battery-powered clock works great away from home. Just don't pick a clock that ticks. Some people find ticking super annoying when they're trying to relax.

Carry Case or Bag

If you're taking your massage show on the road, you'll need simple, portable supplies, and something to carry them in. If you're taking a portable massage table, get a carry case with a strap that slips over your shoulder. Most carry cases have a big pocket for massage supplies and sheets. There are also massage carts if you find the carry case too heavy or unwieldy. If you aren't schlepping a table, a large slouchy "hobo" bag, overnight bag, or reusable grocery bag will hold your massage supplies.

Water

A nice glass of water is very refreshing after a massage—but that's all it is: refreshing. Many people deeply believe that massage releases toxins, and that drinking water afterwards flushes the toxins out, but there's no science to support this.[17] However, massage can be dehydrating because it gets very warm, and may move fluids (which are not themselves toxins) out of the muscles or tissues and into the bloodstream, where they're turned into pee via the kidneys. While drinking water definitely rehydrates the body, it's the kidneys that "release" toxins, and they'll still filter the blood, whether you drink an extra glass of water or not. Toxins are also released in sweat or dispelled—sometimes violently—through the intestines. A glass of water is usually much appreciated after a massage, but whether it's actually *necessary* is questionable. That said, including things just to make someone happy never hurt anyone!

Practice Partner

You can't truly learn the massage techniques and sequences without practicing on a real, live person. Learning massage is like learning to ski or ride a horse. You can read every book there is on the topic, but you won't master those skills until you learn them kinesthetically. Reading is good, but *doing* is mandatory. If your loved one is open to letting you practice on them and learn as you go, and that feels comfortable to you, fine. If not, you'll need a Body Buddy.

A great Body Buddy candidate is someone who can roll with your initial awkwardness or hesitancy without getting annoyed; someone who will laugh with you if you mess up.

---

17. Paul Ingraham, "Why Drink Water After Massage?" PainScience.com, last updated September 1, 2018, https://www.painscience.com/articles/drinking-water-after-massage.php.

And you *will* mess up! That's just part of the learning process. Your Body Buddy should be understanding and patient if you feel nervous or unsure as you're learning to touch, and someone with whom you can get the giggles or lose all your confidence and start over. In other words—someone you feel safe with. A good sense of humor will go a long way as we learn these techniques. Your Body Buddy must also feel comfortable removing their clothing to let you practice. And don't worry—everything that needs to be covered will stay covered!

A Body Buddy is particularly helpful if you don't have a lot of experience with touch, or if you feel hesitant, shy, or uncomfortable about touch. You don't have to launch right into the massage sequences from the start. You can take baby steps with your Body Buddy and just get used to touching someone. Hold a hand, rub the shoulders, or pet the hair. Just get as comfortable with touching that person as you would your cat or dog.

So, how to convince someone to be your Body Buddy? The words "free massage" usually is more than enough. In fact, those words may attract more body buddies than you know what to do with! You can work on one Body Buddy exclusively, or several if you wish. But you must have at least one.

We'll start practicing on your Body Buddy in chapter seven, when we start learning and practicing the various massage sequences. That gives you some time to line up a Body Buddy, or buddies. Going forward, we'll call your Body Buddy simply your "Buddy." That feels nice and cozy.

Notebook

You'll need a blank journal or notebook (plain old spiral bound is perfect) for writing down the massage sequences we'll learn in chapter three. We'll call these notes your "cheat sheets," which you'll use as you learn the sequences for each area, region, and finally, the entire full-body and Sacred Massage sequences. If you use your book, I guarantee it will become saturated with oil. Also, it's just much easier to have it all in one place, and also, the act of writing these sequences down yourself will boost your learning process and memory.

The Niceties

These things, while not absolutely necessary, can really enhance a massage experience.

Air Purifier

If air-borne viruses are an issue or if your loved one suffers from allergies, a standing air purifier with a HEPA filter is great. I prefer the tower kind, which also emit soothing ambient "white noise." If the room is hot or stuffy, an air purifier also moves the air around and provides a gentle, cooling breeze.

Table Warmer

Like a massage table cover, a table warmer has elastic loops at both ends or on the corners to keep it in place while you're working. It's sort of like a big heating pad, and requires an electrical outlet. The warmer goes on the table first, then the table cover, then the sheet. Turn the warmer on about 15 minutes before your session so the table and sheets will be nice and toasty when your loved one settles in. People just *love* the table warmer, particularly in the winter. It makes them go "Ahhhhhh."

Bottle Warmer

During the cold months, cold oil on a nice warm back is a shocker. Electric massage bottle warmers are easily found online. Be sure to loosen the cap on the bottle before warming, or the oil will ooze out of the pump and make a mess. A little hack for warming a bottle is to fill a tall glass of water halfway with hot water (not boiling, just hot from the tap) a couple minutes before your massage session and drop the bottle right into the water. You can microwave massage oil right in the bottle, but remove the pump first if it contains metal, and loosen the cap so it won't explode. Be extra cautious when using a microwave. Only heat in twenty- to thirty-second intervals, take the bottle out, shake it, and test the warmth on the inside of your forearm before using it on someone. Oil doesn't heat evenly in the microwave and can have really hot spots. A bottle warmer will heat to a consistently safe temperature. No matter which heating method you use, always test the oil on yourself before using it on someone else.

Bolsters

Bolsters can be found at any online massage supply website. Unlike pillows, bolsters are easy to clean if oil gets on them, and they're easier to slide in and out when you're propping or supporting an area of the body. Rolled-up towels sometimes get scrunched and wrinkled when you move them. Bolsters come in all sorts of sizes, shapes, and colors.

Body Wedge

If your loved one needs to be propped up while on their back or remain in a reclining position, a body wedge is superb. It provides a long, flat plane and doesn't get all bunchy under the body or flatten out like pillows. Many wedges can be transformed into different shapes and angles, and can double for putting under the knees and elevating the legs. Pick one with a removable, washable cover, but also cover it with a sheet or towel to keep it clean. Side bonus: if you struggle with acid reflux at night, a body wedge will be your new best friend.

Ice Packs, Warm Packs, and Heating Pads

Ice packs, warm packs, and heating pads are useful in massage. A warm pack or heating pad can soften an area before working on it, while some things like tendonitis or swelling actually benefit more from cold than heat. Be careful with both, and don't place them directly on the skin. Cover them with a thin towel or pillowcase. An ice pack should not be left on longer than 20 minutes, with at least a 20-minute interval before using it again. In general, if inflammation or swelling is the underlying issue, it needs cooling down. If the underlying issue is stiffness or tightness, it needs warming up. Therapeutic ice or heat packs are flexible and can be molded around an elbow, shoulder, or other sore spot. You can purchase ice and warm packs online (some packs do both).

Making Do With What You Have

We've covered massage necessities and niceties. However, if all this seems like an overwhelming amount of stuff, or too much expense, be creative and improvise, or make do with what you have. You don't need the most expensive oils or sheets to give a wonderful massage. You can get by just fine with plain old bedsheets and some olive oil, and music playing from your phone. Plain old towels and pillows you already have will do. Just as in magic, it's not the stuff that makes Sacred Massage happen. It's your love and compassion. Your intention. It's *you*.

Chapter 3

Concerns, Contraindications, and Assorted Miscellanea

There are a few things to consider before embarking on your sacred healing journey with your loved one, such as physical or psychological conditions that require additional practice, care, and/or research, and some conditions for which massage might do more harm than good. If you're concerned about anything while massaging your loved one, whether mentioned in this chapter or not—stop. Don't work on that area at all until you get more information and/or speak with a physician—preferably your loved one's.

If your loved one's needs extend beyond simple relaxation and pain relief, find out everything you can about their condition. Get a book. Get several books. Find a support group or someone else experiencing this condition, or who has a loved one with that condition. Google like the wind and find articles and videos—valuable information may be a mere mouse click away. Become an expert on their condition, not to heal or cure it, but to develop a clear understanding of which massage techniques may or may not suit this situation. You may need to alter or eliminate certain tools or techniques, or you may discover that your loved one really needs to level up and see a doctor or physical therapist. If so, you can consult with that professional to see if there's a way to supplement their treatment with your Soothing Touch. Ask which tools and techniques would be beneficial, and which should be avoided. Become a healing partner with your loved one's medical or therapeutic team.

Even with more information and professional consultation, your loved one's needs may be above your pay grade. If their swollen limbs need lymphatic drainage or their tendonitis would respond best to Shiatsu, pass the massage baton on to someone else with more education, experience, and expertise: a licensed massage therapist. And don't feel badly about that. You didn't fail. You made a wise and responsible choice with your loved one's best interests at heart. You might ask that therapist if they're open to teaching you some techniques to help your loved one until their next appointment.

If it turns out that physical massage techniques won't be appropriate for your loved one, you can still do Sacred Massage on most anyone. Your focus would be on the spiritual rather than the physical, and you can still go through the entire Sacred Massage ritual, which we will learn later on. You could substitute gentle, loving palms on the scalp for the massage sequences, or just quietly hold a hand. Even when physical touch must be limited, the Sacred Massage outline remains the same—it happens on the divine, magical level, without any physical massage work actually required. The divine healing and compassion still flow, and the magic still happens.

A Lighter Touch

Every body is not the same, so every massage technique won't work on every person, particularly pressure. Although the sequences we'll cover in part three should be fine for most people, for others, only the gentlest touch is appropriate, and some tools and techniques must be altered or omitted entirely.

Infants and Children

You'll have to completely restructure your tools and techniques to work on an infant. While most infants aren't struggling with neck and shoulder tension from sitting at a computer all day, they do benefit from very light, gentle massage. For simple parent-child bonding, a massage is wonderful. Infant massage can also alleviate colic, improve circulation, help a little one fall asleep, and sometimes soothe a bad case of the crankies.

Finding the pressure for an infant is tricky—it has to be *just* firm enough not to tickle. That "just below ticklish" pressure is "deep" enough. Actually, you really don't use pressure on babies—just slow, light, gentle strokes and caresses with relaxed fingers and fingertips. With babies, you must be a body language expert, because they don't communicate displeasure in words. They stiffen up, turn away, cry, or become cranky. Watch their faces and body movements to assess how you're doing.

Be ultra careful about any oil or lotion you use on a baby. Their brand-new skin is extremely sensitive and delicate. You'll be touching so slowly and gently, you probably don't need to use any oil or lotion at all. The techniques for working on a baby are very different than working on an adult, so you'll need to watch videos and do your homework before massaging your little one.[18] Rather than using a massage table, just sit on the floor with the soles of your feet together, forming a nice diamond shape to keep your infant safe and still.

When working on a toddler or older child, use very light pressure. Simply ask the child as you're working, "Does that feel good?" and let them guide your pressure. Also, you're working on a relatively tiny place, so you'll need to adjust your tools and techniques for that. A flat fist might be way too big to slide down a child's back, but three fingers together might work. You'll probably use your fingers and thumbs much more than your whole hand on a child than on an adult, because they are smaller tools for smaller space.

Massage may help kids with anxiety, getting to sleep, or alleviating leg or foot cramps, and is a wonderfully bonding experience for parents or caretakers and their littles. Massage is a lovely way to help calm and soothe an upset child, and kids experiencing emotional struggles. Just because people are little doesn't mean they don't have powerful and overwhelming emotions. Children also experience grief, anxiety, and fear, and it's even more unsettling for children because they have so very little control over their lives and environment. Rather than belittle or minimize their feelings, softly reassure them as you gently touch: *Everything will be okay…I am here for you…you are safe…"* Notice that I didn't include, "Don't worry," because it's very abrasive and minimizing to tell another person to just stop feeling the way they feel—whether that person is big or small.

At the other end of the emotional scale, if your child gets the giggles from your touch, use your warm, flat palm to gently hold or press that area until they calm down. If the giggles are out of control, just give your child a big, warm hug, tell them you love them, and let it go. Try massage another day.

Fibromyalgia

Fibromyalgia also calls for the lightest touch. A person with fibromyalgia doesn't experience touch in the same way everyone else does. A person with fibromyalgia may experience touch as pain, no matter how gentle. When I'm working on a person with fibromyalgia, I imagine that I'm working on a bubble—I mustn't apply any more pressure than would burst that bubble. I must go extra slowly, and extra, extra gently. It's just one notch above "infant pressure." If that person tells me that something hurts—even something as seemingly gentle and innocuous as spreading oil over the skin—I take their feedback at face

---

18. Amy Zinti, "How to Massage a Baby," Parents.com, last updated October 3, 2005, https://www.parents
.com/baby/care/newborn/how-to-massage-baby/.

value: If they say it hurts, it hurts, end of story. When working on someone with fibromyalgia, you must work within their template of "pain," not your own.

Also, don't be surprised by variations within a condition. There are often exceptions. Even if you *think* you know how to handle a certain condition, your person might tell you otherwise. I once had a woman come for a massage, and she told me she had fibromyalgia; however, she said light touch was extremely irritating to her and she preferred very deep pressure. That was contrary to everything I knew about fibromyalgia! However, *she* was the expert of her experience—not me. I discarded what I knew, and proceeded as she requested.

Bottom line, learn everything you can about the conditions or concerns that apply to your loved one, but don't be rigid. Sure, there are some absolutes, like never applying deep pressure on someone with severe osteoporosis. However, for many other conditions, you may discover that your loved one is the exception to the rule. Let your loved one be the expert on what sort of touch feels best. Just like the customer, your loved one is always right. (As long as their doctor agrees!)

Following are some relatively common conditions you might need to consider before doing massage on your loved one; however, this is definitely not an exhaustive list. If your loved one has a physical or psychological condition and you aren't sure if massage will have a positive or negative effect, don't guess. Consult their physician first.

Autism Spectrum Disorder

Speaking of exceptions to rules, autism spectrum disorder (ASD) will require extra education and experimentation.[19] Any touch, light or deep, may inexplicably trigger a meltdown. That's not bad—it's valuable information: "Don't do that again!" Like fibromyalgia, a person with ASD may not experience touch (or respond to it) in the same way someone without ASD does and, likewise, you must adjust your touch to suit that person. Our own perspective on what touch "should" feel like (and this is true of everyone, not just those with fibromyalgia or ASD) is irrelevant. Soothing Touch is never about us, only about our loved one—even if it doesn't make sense to us.

Oddly enough, touch at the lighter end of the spectrum may be overstimulating for someone with ASD and deeper, firmer touch may work better.[20] Begin a session slowly,

---

19. Michael Regina-Whitely, "Autism and Treatment with Therapeutic Massage." Massage Today, last updated May 29, 2009, https://www.massagetoday.com/articles/13157/Autism-and-Treatment-With-Therapeutic-Massage.

20. Regina-Whitely, "Autism and Treatment with Therapeutic Massage."

keep your voice very low, and use a very limited massage sequence. For some patients, some firm squeezing and holding may be your starting point and that may be the whole session. ASD will require your patience, and guidance from their physician or behavior therapist. Talk to others who have loved ones with ASD and create a massage sequence that suits your loved one.

Arthritis

Lighter touch is preferable for arthritis. Whether rheumatoid arthritis or good old wear and tear, handle arthritic joints with great care. Massage only the tissue around them, and do not attempt to move or manipulate any arthritic joint. Sometimes light squeezing and holding on the arthritic joint feels good. Let your loved one be the guide on how much pressure feel best. Don't attempt to change the position of an arthritic joint or finger. Let it remain as is, and work around it. There should not be any stiff, prickly pain when working on an arthritic joint, and no bending or stretching of that joint. If something hurts, gently stroke that area, and just move on.

Fragile Skin

Be extra gentle when massaging an elderly person. Aging skin can be very loose and fragile, and look like tissue paper, with veins showing prominently. Treat it as if it *is* tissue paper. Keep the touch light, and be extra cautious about gliding and sliding moves. Don't stretch or pull on the skin, which is uncomfortable and might even create bruising. Some extra oil for moisturization might be appreciated on very thirsty skin.

Dementia

According to Ann Catlin's story in Massage Today, "The Role of Massage Therapy in Dementia Care," about one-half of elderly people living in nursing homes or assisted living facilities have dementia. This population suffers from simple lack of touch.

"Lack of human touch is real for the medically frail elder, leading to feelings of isolation, anxiety, poor trust in caregivers, insecurity and decreased sensory awareness," notes Catlin. "Older adults living with serious conditions are often especially receptive to touch. Unfortunately, they are least likely to receive expressive human touch from healthcare providers."[21]

21. Ann Catlin, "The Role of Massage Therapy in Dementia Care," Massage Today, last updated March 16, 2015, https://www.massagetoday.com/articles/15057/The-Role-of-Massage-Therapy-in-Dementia-Care.

For someone with dementia, a slow, soothing hand, foot, or back massage might be appropriate and soothing, and help decrease anxiety and blood pressure, promote better sleep, and reduce some of the more difficult symptoms of dementia, such as agitation, pacing, wandering, and resisting care. Like providing massage to someone with ASD, you'll need to experiment to see what works and what doesn't, and adjust your massage approach accordingly.

Pregnancy

In the first trimester, most women can receive massage lying on their backs or stomachs. However, if morning sickness is an issue, a sitting or reclining position may be more comfortable. A reclining position is also preferable for a woman in her second trimester. Once their pregnancy is showing, make use of reclining and side-lying positions, which are safer and more comfortable than lying flat, faceup or facedown.

For women in their third trimester, lying facedown is out, and even lying faceup should be avoided because the weight of their bellies creates too much pressure on their own organs and circulatory system, which is particularly dangerous if high blood pressure is an issue. In the third trimester, you could use a relining position for only a very short while—maybe to do the shoulders and neck, but the bulk of the session should be done side-lying.

Aching feet are a frequent complaint with pregnant women, and extra time spent there will be appreciated. Some believe that massaging around and just above the ankle may induce contractions or labor. You can gently bypass this area by sliding over it and on up the lower legs. There is also a belief that certain pressure points in the soles of the feet and web of the hand may trigger contractions, so again, slide gently over these areas rather than pressing in or squeezing.[22] Actual scientific evidence for this is lacking,[23] but why not err on the side of caution.

Many pregnant women enjoy and appreciate slow, light, gentle stomach massage (always ask before touching a pregnant woman's stomach), and using some extra soothing moisturizing cream or oil can relieve tight, stretched skin. Never apply pressure to the belly or lean into it. A pregnant woman's lower back can also ache, so spend extra time in the lumbar region and sacrum. Use slow, firm presses in the soft tissue, and lots of kneading.

22. PNSG, "Where NOT to Massage During Pregnancy," PNSG, last updated March 18, 2020, https://pnsingapore.com/blog/where-not-to-massage-during-pregnancy/.

23. Healthline, "How to Safely Get a Massage While Pregnant," Healthline.com, accessed August 27, 2021, https://www.healthline.com/health/pregnancy/where-not-to-massage-a-pregnant-woman#takeaway.

Some pregnancy-related conditions that could be a concern for massage include risk of preterm labor, preeclampsia, high blood pressure, blood clots or a clotting disorder, placenta complications such as placenta previa, and gestational diabetes.[24] If your pregnant loved one has any of these conditions, avoid doing massage until her obstetrician gives you the go-ahead. For more massage tips and techniques that help make a pregnant woman comfortable, while also keeping her and her baby safe, watch some pregnancy massage videos.

Headaches

Headaches are possibly the most common complaint of all. For most headaches, an extended scalp massage feels wonderful—give it lots of gliding with your fingertips, and press the scalp over, across, and around the skull with flat palms. Giving the neck, shoulders, and trapezius extra attention often provides headache relief, because the source of a tension headache can be any or all of the muscles in those areas being chronically tight, or in actual spasm. Many of the upper back and shoulder muscles attach right to the base of the skull. When they tighten, they pull on the skull, straining the scalp muscles. Result: tension headache.

Here are a few methods for relieving headaches:

Web pinch: Firmly pinching the web of the hand between the thumb and index finger can stimulate an acupressure point for headaches. However, the trick is intense pressure. Find that tight spot in the web of the hand, and slowly pinch into it deeper and deeper until your loved one grimaces a little or yelps, "Ouch!" Yes, unlike most other techniques where we will aim for a "delicious ache," this one will hurt. Pinch and hold that spot for at least a minute, and check in with your loved one afterwards to see if there's a positive effect. It may take a couple tries. Some people respond to this acupressure point and sadly, some don't.

Hair pulls: We usually think of having our hair pulled as painful; however, if done correctly, it can relieve a headache. The trick is to grab a lot of hair, in fistfuls, right at the roots. Place the backs of your curved fingers against the scalp, and grab a large amount of hair between your fingers. Make fists, and very slowly squeeze your fists until the middle phalanges of your fingers are resting against the scalp. Hold, release, repeat. Move to another area on the scalp, and repeat. You can also slide

---

24. Healthline, "How to Safely Get a Massage While Pregnant."

the scalp by the hair over the bone while grasping it in your fists—back and forth, and in circles.

Some find hair-pulls amazingly relieving and absolutely love them, and others hate it. It's all about getting an ample amount of hair in your fists, and squeezing slowly. Try this move on yourself before trying it on someone else to learn how much hair to grab and how hard to squeeze for it to feel good rather than painful.

Migraines: Migraines turn headaches into monsters. A scalp massage may provide relief, as can an upper body massage with particular focus on the trapezius, shoulders, neck, jaw, and scalp, particularly if you begin before the migraine is full-blown. If the migraine is going full throttle, a focused upper body massage may be too much extra stimulation. If it's really excruciating, any massage may be experienced as increasing the pain rather than relieving it. Provide touch only as your loved one requests it, and that may mean none at all.

When working on someone in the midst of a migraine, do not play any music, or use anything with scent. Darken the room to only enough light for you to make out shapes—dark enough to go to sleep. Begin by cradling the head with warm, relaxed hands, and become a channel, a river of divine love, compassion, and relief. Breathe slowly, deeply, and effortlessly. Do not talk. Stay completely silent. Just hold. Don't move your hands other than to very gently press with your fingertips and palms. Sit with this for awhile and check in with your loved one for direction—should you continue as you are, or add in some scalp massage? Do as they ask.

Although massage may relieve migraines, if they're an ongoing problem, happening with regularity and frequency, a trip to the doc is in order. Migraines and recurring headaches, severe or not, can be caused by a whole range of things: allergies, eye strain, dehydration, insomnia, and fatigue. And those are the easy ones. There are a lot of not-so-easy causes (and many of them are experienced suddenly, rather than chronically), like tumors, developing brain aneurisms, stroke, or bleeding within the cranium following a severe bump or blow to the head, and those require immediate medical attention.

Some clues that a headache has a serious underlying cause include increasing/escalating headache, vomiting, drowsiness, dizziness, confusion, slurred speech, unequal pupil size, and loss of consciousness, and in particular, slurring of speech and/or weakness or paralysis on one side of the face and/or body. If a severe headache—whether sudden or chronic—is accompanied by any of these symptoms, don't do a massage, don't wait for a doctor's appointment, and don't even go to emergency room unless it's a few blocks away. Call 911. Moments can matter. A lot. Don't take "no" for an answer when these symptoms are present. If your loved one protests, let them, as you're calling 911 anyway.

Allergies

Most of us think of allergies as an annoyance, but certain allergies can be very serious, even lethal, and this is something to consider when choosing your massage oil or lotion. In particular, nut allergies are a concern. If your loved one has nut allergies, *any* nut oil could trigger an allergic reaction. Read the ingredient list carefully. Even if you aren't aware of an allergy, if you start your massage session, and your loved one starts sneezing, coughing, or wheezing, develops a stuffy nose or itchy, red, watery eyes, develops a rash, hives, or other sign of skin irritation, stop immediately and contact their physician for advice. Don't take it lightly. Severe allergic reactions can be deadly, and can escalate quickly.

If your loved one has difficulty breathing, develops swelling of the lips, tongue, throat, eyes, or face, starts vomiting, develops low blood pressure or faints, this sort of severe reaction is called *anaphylaxis*, and is an immediate medical emergency. Call 911. Anaphylaxis symptoms can occur within seconds of exposure to an allergen and become life-threatening quickly. This is not something you can handle yourself. An EpiPen can buy you some time to get to the emergency room, but the only acceptable emergency treatment for anaphylaxis is an epinephrine injection from an emergency responder or medical professional.[25] If your loved one is prone to allergic reactions, make sure you know the signs of anaphylaxis and what to do,[26] and always have an EpiPen handy. Don't attempt to diagnose and treat the symptoms yourself. If you aren't sure whether the allergic reaction is severe or not, err on the side of caution and let a doctor decide.

If you want to be extra cautious about potential allergies, rub your massage oil or lotion onto the inside of your loved one's forearm and wait an hour to see if there's a reaction.

25. Parul Kothari, "Epinephrine is the Only Effective Treatment for Anaphylaxis," Harvard Health Publishing, last updated July 9, 2020, https://www.health.harvard.edu/blog/epinephrine-is-the-only-effective-treatment-for-anaphylaxis-2020070920523.

26. Jennifer Warner, "When is an Allergic Reaction an Emergency?" EverydayHealth.com, last updated April 15, 2014, https://www.everydayhealth.com/hs/anaphylaxis-severe-allergy-guide/allergic-reaction-emergency/.

Varicose Veins

Varicose veins occur when the valves inside the veins that help pump blood back to the heart work inefficiently or sometimes not at all. This causes a backflow of blood in the legs and impairs circulation. The veins can stretch and create unsightly bumpy ropes just under the skin. However, veins deeper inside the leg can also fail, and cause the legs to feel heavy and tired. Sometimes swelling in the feet and ankles occurs. The concern for massaging over varicose veins is that blood clots can occur, particularly at the valve sites, and massage can dislodge them. If your loved one has varicose veins with blood clots, do not work these areas at all. It should be okay to elevate their legs on a cushion while you massage other areas. In fact, elevating the legs is often recommended as a way of alleviating discomfort and poor circulation due to varicose veins.

If blood clots aren't an issue, light massage on the legs may alleviate some of the discomfort and swelling. Deep pressure should never be applied to areas with varicose veins; massage should be light and remain near the surface. When working over varicose veins, gentle glides in the direction of the heart can assist circulation. If there is pain or redness on a varicose vein, avoid this area.[27]

Be aware that while light massage might offer relief for someone with varicose veins, it won't make a significant improvement or serve as a cure. The condition is typically treated medically, where the veins are either cauterized and dissolved, or removed surgically, and managed by wearing compression stockings.[28] In an abundance of caution, get clearance from your loved one's physician before working over varicose veins.

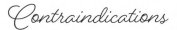

Contraindications

Beyond the conditions that necessitate further learning or consultation with a professional, or immediate medical intervention, some conditions are a "hard stop" for massage. These are called "contraindications," and they mean one thing: Don't. Even for a professional massage therapist, there are several things that are beyond their scope of practice, and belong in a physician's care.

27. Medical Massage Therapy, "Varicose Veins Massage," MassageTherapyReference.com, accessed July 22, 2022, https://www.massagetherapyreference.com/varicose-veins-massage/.

28. Vein & Vascular Institute editor, "Does Massage Help Varicose Veins," Vein & Vascular Institute, accessed January 15, 2020, https://www.veinvascular.com/vein/does-massage-help-varicose-veins/.

Amongst the contraindications for massage are: bleeding disorders, skin rashes, burns, healing wounds, deep vein thrombosis, blood clots, deep or severe bruising, infections, fever, contagious diseases, severe osteoporosis, and taking blood-thinning medications.

Massage is also contraindicated for broken bones, or fresh muscle, tendon, or soft tissue tears, injuries, or recent surgery. Anything broken or torn cannot be "fixed" with more manipulation or movement. That area needs to just be left alone to heal. With guidance from a physician, ice, a heating pad, or elevation may assist healing—but massage won't. Give it time.

In the case of severe burns or rashes, or any condition where your loved one can't be touched *at all*, you might consider learning Reiki or Healing Touch, which do not need to include physical touch. Substitute those techniques for the Sacred Massage sequences you'll be learning later on, and rather than touching your loved one, sit next to them (or as close as possible), face your palms toward them, ground, center, and focus, and channel divine healing and magical energy toward them that way. You can still perform the magical Sacred Massage sequences mentally, in your mind and follow them step-by-step without making any physical contact at all. Your presence and devotion will still provide comfort and reduce stress. When away from your loved one, make use of magical practices and ritual to implement and manifest healing and relief.

To the official list of contraindications, I have a few of my own: fever, cough or sneezing that produces any fluid that isn't clear, or any other cold or flu symptoms not caused by seasonal allergies. Seasonal allergies, while certainly a misery, aren't contagious, and a relaxing massage may be helpful, if you don't mind occasional sneezing and have plenty of tissues handy.

If your loved one lives with you and has cold or flu symptoms, you've already been exposed, so whether or not you want to provide some Soothing Touch depends on whether or not you are also developing symptoms and feel up to doing a massage or not. That said, increase circulation just helps the virus circulate further. Stick to gently holding, touching, and pressing. No gliding or sliding. Someone with a fever might be soothed by a cool cloth on their forehead and some gentle stroking of the hair, but that's probably enough Soothing Touch for the moment. A partner with an upset stomach or intestinal issues may appreciate your warm palm resting on their stomach, and long, smooth gliding strokes elsewhere. When it's someone who lives with you, use your best judgment if your loved one is under the weather. If you have even the slightest niggles of concern, sorry, you'll have to disappoint them. They'll have to settle for some warm tea and a blankie until they feel better.

If it's you who is developing cold or flu symptoms, don't do any massage on others. You'll expose them to whatever you have, and you will also not be at your best, physically, spiritually, or magically.

Contagious Disease

If COVID or some other contagious virus is a concern, follow whatever public health guidelines are in place. If your loved one is in a hospital or assisted living, you must follow the rules for that facility. If there's an outbreak of significant concern, unless you and your loved one live together, you must wear a KN95 mask during your session. Not a cheap-o knockoff—the real deal. Purchase them from a medical supplier, because your life and your loved one's may depend on that mask doing its job.

Other precautions when contagious viruses are a concern include sanitizing non-porous surfaces (such as your massage table), washing all sheets and blankets in hot water after each use, washing your hands before and after working on someone, and working in a well-ventilated area or even outside if possible. Get a HEPA air filter with an ultraviolet light that will kill viruses. Also, regular viral testing (for you *and* your loved one) are good safety precautions.

I know that some people aren't comfortable with vaccines, but I'll share my position: I stay current on all vaccines and boosters, not only because I don't want to spread any virus to someone else, but also because if I catch a cold or the flu, let alone something worse, I'm unable to work until I'm completely symptom-free. Nobody wants to hear their massage therapist sniffling or coughing during their special hour. In my opinion, staying current on vaccines is the most compassionate and responsible thing you can do when interacting with others.

And Now, a Little Nagging

Before we dive into part two, there are a few things you need to do to make your Sacred Massage a pleasant experience for your loved one. They may seem small, but they really do matter.

Trim Those Nails!

My first day in massage school, the instructor told us, "If the white on your fingernails is showing, they're too long." And then, she lined us up and inspected every hand. Those who didn't pass inspection were instructed to trim their nails before returning to class the following day, when we'd start practicing massage techniques on each other.

Before placing your hands on anyone else, trim or file your nails, with as little white showing as possible. Make sure every edge and corner is filed smooth. You can test this by running your fingernails over stretchy fabric, like nylons, tights, or yoga pants. If they catch, file again. It's astonishingly uncomfortable and startling to suddenly feel a sharp or jagged fingernail on your bare skin during a massage. Worse still, you could cause a nasty scratch or even draw blood. Drawing blood is definitely the ultimate party foul for massage! Besides your fingernails, trim off any rough or ragged hangnails, and use an emery board to sand down callouses or rough spots. Ragged hangnails scratch the skin too, and interrupt relaxation.

In between sessions, get into the habit of maintaining your hands as conduits of divine healing energy. Get into the habit of using hand lotion after washing your hands and before bedtime. If someone was touching your bare skin, you'd like to feel smooth, soft hands—not nasty, crusty old lobster claws with jagged nails and rough callouses. Take care of your hands like the sacred, magical tools they are!

Wash Those Hands!

You must wash your hands before every massage session, and also afterwards. Make sure your nails are clean too. Nothing says *"yuck"* like a line of gray scum under your fingernails. Besides simply looking more presentable, your hands and nails must be clean before you touch someone so you don't pass along any communicable diseases or viruses. If your hands are dirty and you touch your loved one's hands, and then they scratch their nose or eyes, you may pass along a virus. Conversely, just in case your loved one wasn't diligent about washing their hands before you begin your session, you don't want to pick up a virus from them. After your session, immediately go wash your hands while your loved one gets dressed, and use that washing time to thank your hands for all that divine, magical work they've done, and cleanse them of any unwanted energy.

Warm Them Up!

Besides dirty hands, there's another "hand party foul" for massage: cold hands. Sadly, some of us are afflicted with icy hands (me!), particularly in the wintertime, and nothing is more shocking and more un-relaxing than frosty fingers on your nice, warm back or sides. You can get microwavable hand-warmers to wear before your session, rub your hands briskly before starting, or do extra warmup moves over the sheet to get your own blood flowing before touching your loved one. Using warmed massage oil can offset cold hands a bit. When all else fails, and my hands are still too cold, I warn my clients and apologize in advance, and tell them, "Imagine this is a cool breeze, soothing all your inflammation." It seems to help a bit. I also reassure them that, not to worry, my hands will warm right up after a couple minutes. If my hands are really chilly, I also start at the neck and shoulders while warming up, rather than mid-back, as these areas are less reactive to a sudden shock of cold.

Take Off That Jewelry!

Jewelry, whether on you or your loved one, can get in the way, leave a nasty scratch, or in the case of dangly earrings, be quite dangerous. Your loved one needs to remove earrings, bracelets, necklaces, and their watch before a massage session. Rings should come off too, but you can work around wedding rings if your loved one is uncomfortable removing it. Provide a little cup or dish to hold jewelry during your session.

As for you, the rings must come off, and that includes a wedding band that has stones or protrusions. I promise your marriage won't dissolve if you do. If it's a flat, smooth band, you get away with that if you're very careful. If you just cannot bring yourself to remove your wedding ring, you'll have to be abundantly cautious not to scratch your loved one. Everything else must go, and that includes bracelets and watches, or anything around your wrists. If you're wearing a pendant that's so long that it might touch your loved one as you work, tuck it into the neckline of your shirt.

Help the Heart!

In part three, we'll be learning all sorts of moves and techniques in all sorts of places, but one is worth emphasizing: When massaging limbs (arms and legs), you apply pressure to push your strokes toward the heart, and release and start over, or gently slide on the way back. This is because massage aids circulation in the limbs, and the goal is to assist the blood on its return to the heart, particularly through the legs. Blood goes in the direction of the heart on its return, and away from the heart as it is pumped out. We want to move in the direction that assists the heart, rather than working against it.

Don't Push It!

One of the massage techniques we'll be learning is pushing and pressing into various soft tissue. However, there are some things you must never push, press, or lean into: the spine, the eyes, the front of the neck/throat, the sides of the neck immediately next to the throat, the sternum, and the belly/abdominal cavity. With the exception of the eyes, which you should avoid entirely, it's okay to lightly slide oil over these areas without using any pressure if your loved one finds it soothing; however, all of these areas are usually avoided in massage.

Wash Those Sheets!

If you use oil or lotion during your Sacred Massage, you must wash them after *every* use. Sure, it *seems* like you should be able to use them more than once, because after all, you sleep on your bed sheets for much longer—several days, maybe even weeks. However, you aren't putting layer after layer of oil on your bed sheets. Even though you only used your massage sheets for an hour, they're going to get a lot of oil on them. The longer it sets, the harder it is to remove. If the oil sets for too long, it will become rancid and smell awful. Worse yet, a buildup of rancid oil can be a fire hazard in the dryer.

After each use, wash your sheets in hot water and rinse in hot or warm water—not cold. Cold water just hardens oils back up again. Don't use fabric softener, because that's just another layer of chemicals on top of the oil. If you just can't bring yourself to forego fabric softener, pick an unscented one and only use about a tablespoon, rather than the capful the manufacturer recommends. Unscented detergent is also preferable for massage sheets.

Even if you wash your massage sheets faithfully, they can still become saturated with oil over time and rancid smelling. Once that stench sets in, it's difficult to get it out. Presoaking in hot water with a half-gallon of white vinegar for an hour, followed by washing regularly in hot water, will help. A professional-grade detergent specifically designed to remove oil can help prevent oil buildup. If your sheets still smell rancid after trying these methods, cut them up and use them as rags to wash your car. Don't subject your loved one to that horrid smell.

As for blankets, if you're careful, you can just wash them as needed. They don't typically get a lot of oil on them. But if they get *that* smell—donate them to a veterinary hospital or animal rescue center. That said, animals may not even want to lie on them.

Be Quiet!

Massage is a meditative process for both giver and receiver, and just as in an actual meditation, if you're yammering on about what you want to make for dinner, or who pissed you off that morning, or what the talking heads on the evening news had to say, your focus is scattered all over the place, rather than on your loved one. That serene, spiritual meditative experience just dissolves into the ether. Worse yet, all that yakking pretty much destroys your loved one's opportunity to sink into relaxation.

My two hard and fast rules regarding conversation during a massage are "Speak only when necessary" and "Speak when spoken to." Period.

Unless.

There are some people really do enjoy chatting during their massage. In that case, I have another hard and fast rule: "It's not about me." In other words, it's *their* hour, not mine. If someone wants to chat, then we chat. I follow their lead. If they go quiet for a bit, I mirror that energy and go quiet too. I will say this, however—while you could still do massage techniques while chatting, all that talking and distraction *will* negatively affect a Sacred Massage experience. Talking interferes with channeling divine, magical energy, just like static on the radio. The communication becomes garbled and difficult. Talking prevents you from easing into your quiet, calm, clear place and ruins your concentration for doing your best divine, magical work. Even so, if your loved one is a Chatty Cathy, it's still *their* massage. Let them chat. Just do your best. It might not be sacred, but if it makes your loved one feel better, it's still worthwhile and beneficial.

Keep It Covered, and Don't Touch!

In order to respect and be sensitive to your loved one's sense of modesty, certain areas of the body, such as the genitals and breasts, must remain covered with a massage sheet at all times. Anything under that sheet is off-limits. It should go without saying, but I'm saying it anyway: Sexual touch or activity of any kind is a hard stop in massage. It's a big, fat "NO." Aside from the glutes, if it's something that needs to be covered at a public swimming pool, it's something that can't be touched in a massage session. Genitals and breasts are never to be exposed, or touched. Ever. (Unless your loved one is also your consenting partner, but that's a topic for an entirely different book.)

It's Ultimately for the Best

I know, I know … this chapter was kind of a drag. But you need be aware of these precautions and conditions before providing Sacred Massage to your loved one. These things may not be concerns at the moment and you may never deal with them at all. However, if they pop up, you'll recognize them and know how to respond.

Always approach every condition and situation with love and compassion in your heart, and concern for your loved one's health and happiness above all else. These are the cornerstones of Sacred Massage.

PART TWO

The Spiritual and Magical Side of Massage

Chapter 4

Touch Is Spiritual

In massage school, we learned all about bones and bodies, and muscles and tendons, and what to do with them. We mastered many techniques for easing tension and promoting relaxation in the body, but there was one thing missing: spirituality. Maybe the topic of spirituality leaned a little too close to religion and, like politics, discussing religion in a mixed group of people can trigger conflict—the last thing you want in a massage class. So, of *course* we're going to talk about it here!

If the mention of spirituality already triggered your anxiety, relax. Everything will be okay. There will be no proselytizing, and no criticism. I'll share my own spiritual angle so you know where I'm coming from, but I'm not going to persuade you to share in my beliefs. Wherever I use my own spirituality and mention my preferred deities, you can swap in your own. You can use my template, but customize it to your own belief system. If your spiritual beliefs lean closer to agnosticism or even atheism, substitute whatever works for you—maybe nature or love and compassion. But we need some sort of spiritual component to elevate a typical massage to a Sacred Massage. Without any spiritual element, massage might still be relaxing and beneficial, but it can be so much more.

Even if you're already committed to a certain spiritual path, I believe that being open to other spiritual or religious viewpoints has value. I cherry-pick from other belief systems and practices all the time, but I do so with respect for the culture from which they came. If a belief, technique, or approach feels true and valuable in my own heart, I keep it. If not, I take a pass. You can consider different perspectives, and take them or leave them, or include particular practices that feel meaningful and worthwhile to you, but always be sensitive to the culture from which they came. If it's a culture or religion other than your own, be respectful of that root source. If you feel a deep attraction to a culture that isn't your own, learn about the culture and deepen your understanding, and treat it with respect. Don't adopt it as your own and, in particular, don't present yourself as a member of that culture or attempt to profit from it—this is "cultural appropriation," which is insensitive and disrespectful.

Being open to spiritual or religious viewpoints different from your own can help you be more sensitive to a loved one that holds different spiritual perspectives than your own. For example, if your loved one is a devoted Christian, you might use different terminology, like "God" instead of "the universe," or "angels" instead of "goddesses" or "spirit guides." When you're doing massage, sacred or otherwise, it is *always* about what the other person needs—not you.

My Sacred Massage Path

Incorporating spirituality and divinity into massage wasn't something I learned in massage school, or in any of my continuing education classes. It was touched upon in Reiki and Ayurveda, but not in any deep, comprehensive way—more like a footnote. The spiritual component of my massage practice developed organically on its own. It blossomed from that experience I mentioned, cradling a person's head in my hands, when I had an epiphany about how sacred and precious this experience actually was. At just that moment, the Namaste mantra drifted through my mind: "The divine in me honors the divine in you." This phrase comes from the Sanskrit language and was found in ancient Hindu texts called the "Vedas," but the phrase has become common in many situations, and is the customary blessing at the end of many American yoga classes. So, the spiritual component of Sacred Massage began at this point—blessing and honoring my clients with a Namaste at the end of each session.

Over time, the spiritual element of my massage sessions evolved organically, bit by bit. I created my own personal blessing that I bestow on each client: "Be well and be peaceful, beautiful person." After taking a Reiki class and being given the beginning Reiki symbol called Cho Ku Rei from the Reiki master who taught the class, I blended that into each session too.[29]

---

29. Vlad Dimancea, "Cho Ku Rei: Explore the Untapped Potential of A Versatile Reiki Symbol," ReikiScoop, accessed January 3, 2022, https://reikiscoop.com/cho-ku-rei-reiki-symbol/.

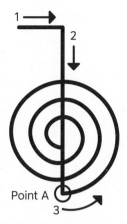

FIGURE 1: CHO KU REI SYMBOL

Reiki is considered as much a spiritual practice as a massage modality, and enjoys dual citizenship with the magical community as well. Reiki employs three sacred symbols, including Cho Ku Rei, which is learned during the first level of training. In traditional Reiki, it is believed that one must be "attuned" to Reiki by a master, and be given the symbol first-person rather than learning it from a book. In my Reiki class, we learned that the sacred symbols were passed personally from Reiki master to Reiki master down through time, keeping the sacred energy intact. Although I love learning from books, I tend to agree on this point. It's entirely more meaningful to go through the Reiki attunement ceremony and be granted the symbol than it is to read words on a page. I included the symbol here so you can understand what I'm referring to, but as I said—if you want to use this symbol, take a Reiki class, become attuned, and receive the symbol from a master. Reiki is a peaceful, gentle supplement to Sacred Massage, and helps one develop energetic sensitivity. A Reiki therapist manipulates and clears energy fields, imbalances, and blockages. It's safe for anyone, even the most fragile people.

I don't focus on Reiki in my massage practice, mainly because I strongly prefer actual physical touch to energy work. However, the Cho Ku Rei blessing has become part of my finishing sequence. While seated behind the client's head, I trace the Cho Ku Rei with my chin above the length of the body while envisioning the symbol, and then transmit its blessing. Cho Ku Rei is a cleansing symbol, associated with protection and activating energy. It brings a gentle effervescence to the end of a massage session, leaving the person feeling clear and refreshed.

My Own Winding Spiritual Path

Right about the time I discovered massage, I randomly and serendipitously toddled onto the Pagan path, where I discovered a world of spiritual practices and deities that suited my values, beliefs, and massage practice. Although there are many specific groups, called "traditions" or "paths" in the Pagan world, I'm not aligned with a particular tradition or pantheon. I describe myself as a "garden-variety Pagan," free to craft my own spiritual path and practices. I'm a spiritual hunter-gatherer. If a deity or practice resonates with me, I put it in my spiritual basket. If not, I just nod, say "thanks," and move on.

I was raised agnostic, without any religious practices or discussions at all, but looking back, I realize I'd always been Pagan, but just didn't have a vocabulary or frame of reference for it. I was just born that way—a wild child, more at home out in nature and with animals than I was indoors or with people. I had a brief excursion into Christianity after marrying into a very small town that didn't have much else to offer in the way of socializing, and this experience took me way out into the spiritual weeds, far from my own true self. After a decade or so of wearing a spiritual costume, I walked away from church and set out to find a spiritual path that felt genuine to me. I found it in Paganism. *This* is where I belong. No pretending, no costumes—just little old genuine me.

I share my spiritual evolution so we're clear on where I'm coming from, and also to suggest that you can also change the spiritual path you're on if it's unfulfilling or feels disingenuous. Sacred Massage requires spiritual honesty. That's the only way to open up to divine healing, love, and compassion. Putting Spirit in a box never works.

Activity
INVITING DEITY INTO MASSAGE

There are many ways to involve deity in your massage sessions. Some are internal and private, and your loved one may not even be aware of what you're doing or attracting. Some loved ones may really appreciate knowing that you're making a special call to a certain deity for them, and you can tell them as you begin that, "I am inviting Kuan Yin (for example) to be with us." If your loved one prefers a more traditional spiritual path, they might find it soothing if you invite the healing touch of angels into your session.

Inviting deity into your own heart, mind, and spirit as you begin a massage session creates a shift within you. Before even touching your loved one, let your healing deity touch you. Take a moment to be still and quiet, envisioning that deity and inviting it into your heart and mind. You might repeat a mantra associated with that deity, or create one of your own, like "May the love and compassion of Tara be within me." If you get distracted, frustrated, or challenged during your session, you can use that mantra to regain your focus and spiritual balance.

Externally, there are many ways to represent divine energy in massage and reinforce your relationship with a deity or divine energy. If you're working in your own space, it's simple: Place images and prompts in that space to reinforce your divine connection and serve as a prompt for remaining in a peaceful, compassionate space while you work. If you're working in someone else's space, your relationship a special deity is totally portable. If you'd like to enhance it with external prompts, bring small images or figurines of your chosen deity, or wear clothing or jewelry that reinforces your connection and keeps you in your spiritual groove.

Activities
DEVELOPING A DIVINE RELATIONSHIP

Relationships form from within, even when your partner is a manifestation of divine energy. Here are some ways to develop and strengthen your internal spiritual relationship with divine energy and deity:

Meditation

Claim some quiet time when you won't be disturbed, and find a comfortable spot, sitting or lying down. Breathe slowly and deeply, into and out of your belly button. Notice the steadiness and safety of whatever surface is supporting you. Breathe. If thoughts intrude, acknowledge them: *That's a thought.* Then mentally swipe them away and return to focus on your breath.

When you feel still and calm, ask the universe to introduce you to the divine energy or deity you need. Request the honor of their presence. You may experience a feeling, sensation, word, color, or image. These are clues for helping you connect with a deity that is interested in you. Think or say a mantra to strengthen that relationship such as "May we provide comfort and healing through touch." Thank that deity for their presence. Return your focus to your breathing, open your eyes, and rejoin the space around you. If you're unsure about who that deity was, remain open to any more clues about that deity's identity. Watch for seren-dipities and symbols. It may be that deity waving "hello!"

This simple meditation can be done any time you feel the need. Just follow the pattern: Breathe, become still, invite deity, connect, think or say a mantra, express gratitude, breathe, return.

Prayer

Most people are familiar with praying, particularly to God (Allah, Spirit, the universe, or whichever name you prefer for that divine entity). Often in prayer, you speak directly to that deity, sometimes out loud. If you prefer prayer to meditation, this is perfectly fine. Approach it as you would meditation: Quiet your mind, open your heart, and let the words flow from there. If you prefer to pray in a particular fashion according to your own spiritual beliefs, do so. Prayer strengthens your relationship with Spirit. If your loved one is deeply religious, praying together before a massage session may be greatly appreciated.

Study

When you find a deity that resonates with you, immerse yourself in learning more so you can deepen your understanding and strengthen your bond. Some deities seem pretty straightforward, such as the Greek goddess Iris, who creates a rainbow as she brings her water-filled urn to the gods, while others are quite complex, such as the Celtic goddess Brigid, a "Jill-of-all-trades." Brigid can do anything, from poetry to protecting farm animals to forging metal. You could spend a lot of time just studying a single aspect of Brigid's skills and talents.

The more you learn about your deity, the stronger your bond will be. You'll also discover all sorts of lore and symbols associated with that deity, which may inspire you as you decorate your massage space or create an altar or focal point. If you discover a relatively obscure deity that you just love, you may have to put a little extra effort into your exploration and learning, such as visiting a library or arranging an appointment to speak with an expert on the topic, like a college professor or clergy. A world of information about deities is easily found online, such as college or university websites, well-known cultural or historical websites like National Geographic or Encyclopedia Britannica, or multi-faceted spiritual websites like Patheos.com. There are even entire websites devoted just to a particular deity.

Reinforcing Your Divine Relationship

You can reinforce your relationship with a deity with external prompts that bring that deity to mind during the course of your day. You don't want to limit your relationship to just prayer or meditation—you want it to be part of your life. Here are some suggestions for strengthening your divine relationship:

Symbols

Choose a symbol associated with your favorite deity and place it where you'll see it every day. You can draw or paint your own image, take photos in nature or museums, purchase figurines or items associated with that deity, or create your own items yourself. For example, the Egyptian goddess Bastet, who is a protectress of women, children, and babies, is also famously associated with cats and sometimes depicted with the head of a cat or entirely as a cat. Placing images of cats in your home can prompt you to think of Bastet, and maybe even to thank her for bringing protection into your life. The more present your healing deity is in your daily life, the more meaningful it will be to include that deity in your Sacred Massage sessions.

You can also wear jewelry or symbols, or carry items, that prompt a reminder and connection to your deity. It might be a symbol on a pendant, or a particular stone in your pocket. Maybe it's a symbol of your own spiritual practice or religion, such as a cross or Star of David. Maybe it's a T-shirt with a certain phrase or symbol that inspires the energy or emotion you associate with that deity, like a lotus flower for Kuan Yin or the Ohm symbol, which represents the divine, infinite energy of the entire universe. Maybe it's all of the above! You can never over-reinforce your connection to divine compassion, love, and healing.

These sorts of symbols and items are also easily transported if you'll be working on a loved one away from your home.

Meditation Beads

Meditation beads (also called prayer beads, worry beads, misbaha, malas, or rosary beads) are a loop of beads held in one's hand while meditating or praying. Each bead is pulled through the fingers one at a time as a particular word, chant, or mantra is spoken or thought. Meditation beads are used in many religions, including Catholicism, Islam, Hinduism, and Buddhism, and each has their own name for the beads as well as the number of beads on the loop. There are usually 108 meditation beads on a loop, plus a "stopper" or "Guru" bead that gives you a tactile clue that you've finished your meditation. (The number "108" has spiritual significance in Buddhism.) Meditation beads are treated as sacred items, and may be kept on altars or in special boxes, or even worn as a necklace. Wearing them or placing them in your massage space can be calming and centering, and spiritually reinforcing.

In Shannon Yrizarry's beautiful little book *Modern Guide to Meditation Beads*, she explains the symbology and cultural history of mala beads, as well as many meditations or mantras to enhance this form of meditation. She also explains how to make your own string, which you could dedicate to the healing deity you've chosen for your massage sessions. You could also create or dedicate a string to simply reinforce values that enhance massage, such as compassion, peace, serenity, love, and healing.

Deity Altars

Altars serve a variety of purposes, which we will discuss in more detail in the next chapter. For honoring or reinforcing your relationship with your special deity, you can create a special altar for enhancing your divine relationship or to serve as a visual prompt that reminds you of that deity's divine healing energy while doing a massage or just as you go about your day. It can be a quiet meditation spot, or a place to speak or pray to that deity—your own personal temple to spend time together.

I have altars all over my house for all sorts of purposes, but in my massage office, I have one just for the Chinese Buddhist goddess Kuan Yin, who inspires compassion and a will to relieve pain, tension, and stress. She is my chosen healing deity and her altar sits upon a little table, and features a small white figurine of her, meditating while seated upon a lotus, which is one of her symbols. The altar is adorned with rose quartz, clear quartz, a crystal lotus, and a string of Swarovski crystals scattered at her feet. It is illuminated by a little lamp with a pink shade that casts gentle, warm light over her and her altar, as well as the massage area. This is the only light I use during a massage. Part of my massage ritual preparation is to light the lamp and welcome Kuan Yin into my heart, my hands, and the session. I ask her to let her compassion flow right through my hands. When the session is over, I thank her for her presence and participation, and turn the light off, leaving her to meditate in her special place.

This is just one example of what a deity altar might look like, and how you might use it. Your own altar will be a creation that represents your own divine relationship. There's no "right" way to create a deity altar, other than to express your appreciation and connection to that deity. It can be simple or elaborate, or somewhere in between, and don't feel shy about making it beautiful. Deities being deities, there's no such thing as "over the top" for them. Pour all your love, appreciation, admiration, and devotion into your altar, commune with your deity there, bring offerings of what they might like—treats, music, flowers—and *feel* that altar come alive with divine energy. You can adorn the altar with shells, crystals, incense, candles, and images of that deity, as well as symbols or items associated with that deity.

If you prefer an altar aligned with your own established spiritual or religious practice, use items associated with that, such as symbols, images, and holy books or quotes. If you prefer to attract a certain type of energy rather than honor a deity as part of your Sacred Massage, use images, symbols, or items that capture your intent, such as hearts, the sun or moon, flowers, shells, trees, or the ocean. You could even include images of actual people who represent kindness, healing, and compassion to you: Mother Theresa, or your favorite aunt, or Oprah, or your doctor.

Exploring Deity and the Divine

There are thousands upon thousands of deities associated with every country and culture spanning the globe, some ancient and archaic, some still quite relevant to modern life and included in everything from religious devotion to rituals to celebrations. To mention them all would be an exhaustive, multi-volume project, and also rather redundant, as there's already a sea of information about most any deity only a mouse-click or library visit away. Additionally, we aren't seeking a comprehensive exploration of deity. Rather, we're narrowing our focus to a sampling of deities that particularly lend themselves to compassion and healing in Sacred Massage.

The All Encompassing

We'll begin our divine exploration at the very top: God. This divine, eternal flow of energy, life, and creation is known by many other names, including Allah, Yahweh, the All, Spirit, the Great Spirit, Source, or the universe. People have different perceptions of that divine energy based upon their religious or cultural upbringing, and call it a particular name, but, it's the same divine energy. For example, an "apple" is "mela" in Italian, "pomme" in French, and "manzana" in Spanish. People speaking different languages use a different word for the same thing. The particular label we humans attach to the apple has no effect on it. It still is what it is—which is essentially how God is said to have defined themself in the Old Testament: "I am." In other words, "Your question of who I am or what to call me makes no sense, human. I'm not even a *who*. I just *am*." I love that: "I am existence itself." Eternal, vibrant, without form, and present in everyone and everything throughout the universe. This description works for me. I usually refer to that divine energy as Spirit or the universe, rather than "God."

If you're drawn to interacting directly with that overarching divine energy, without any spiritual "middleman," then by all means do so. You can be wildly creative in an altar to honor that Source, because it's so broad and all-encompassing. Many healers channel love and energy directly from Source, without any deities involved at all. Many Indigenous people in the United States, for example, speak directly to the Great Spirit in their spiritual and religious practices.

"God" is all, and it's "all good," no matter what you label It.

The Goddess

In many Pagan traditions, the Goddess is central to worship, ritual, spiritual practices, and traditions. Not all of them define the Goddess in the same way. That's one of the beauties of a Pagan life: There's no central authority figure to decree the right and wrong way to do anything, no Pagan Pope. As a Pagan, you are your own authority figure, free to choose how to express and practice your spirituality. Worship, veneration, and exaltation of the Goddess extend to the outskirts of the Pagan world, into New Age practices and traditions, and lately She can be found even in mundane circles and celebrated as divine feminine energy.

I define the Goddess as the eternal, living energy of the planet on which we live. She is all the life, plant and animal, all the seasons, all the land and water, all the weather, and energetically connected with the moon and its phases, and even the times of day. She is the "All" of our earth. Some Pagans equate the Goddess with God (or whatever they call the divine energy of the universe), but for me, there's a difference. God is "All" of the entire universe, while the Goddess is the heartbeat and breath of our tiny, precious blue planet, spinning in that vast sea of celestial bodies, dark matter, and dark energy. Earth is fragile, precious, and rare, so my relationship with the Goddess comes from my deep appreciation of our living planet. For me, protecting the planet is equivalent to honoring the Goddess, and before I gush about this and get way out into the spiritual weeds, let's just pull me up here and summarize that the Goddess might be a comfortable fit for connecting to divine energy if you love nature and the environment, and don't want to walk a particular religious path. Like "God," the Goddess has a vast and wide span. We may be of this spiritual tradition or that, but we are all humans living on this earth and owe it—and Her—some respect and appreciation. You can channel your love for the Goddess, the earth, nature, and the environment right into your Sacred Massage, right toward your loved one.

Healing Deities and Icons

The following list of deities and icons, in alphabetical order, come from a variety of cultures, spiritualities, and religious practices, but they all have one thing in common: healing or compassion, or both, amongst their most prominent attributes. You don't have to stick to just one, but if you're brand new to deity, it might be simpler to pick one that jumps out and catches your fancy. You can always invite more deities into your life later on. If you're attracted to deities from different pantheons, that's okay too. Deities can coexist peacefully with one another and become a divine team—your own personal pantheon. My own pantheon is quite eclectic: Roman, Greek, Egyptian, Celtic, Wiccan, and Buddhist; one big happy family! Some people view deities as specific, unique divine entities, while others view them as expressions, facets, or manifestations of one, single divine energy. I'm of the latter category. I view each deity as a beautiful, colored facet on an immense divine disco ball. Each facet is illuminated by one, single light: Spirit.

If you enter into a relationship with a deity and realize it just isn't clicking, it's not a lifelong commitment. Respectfully thank that deity for all that they taught you, bid them a grateful farewell, and move on.

Here's a small sampling of healing and compassionate deities—and individuals—from a variety of pantheons and religions. There's much more to discover about each one. Each description is just a smidge of information to tickle your interest and imagination, and possibly point you in a particular direction:

> **Airmed/Airmid (Celtic):** Healing with herbs was Airmed's forte. She is of the Tuatha de Danaan, an ancient divine Celtic tribe. She is known for hidden wisdom that can only be accessed through intuition, and was a "master Druid," honoring plant and tree spirits to connect with their knowledge.[30] She is portrayed as healing selflessly and altruistically, not for fame or profit. She is often likened to the Norse goddess, Eir. If you wish to enhance your own selfless, altruistic desire to provide healing, and you're drawn to natural, herbal remedies, Airmed might inspire you.

---

30. Claudia Merrill, "Airmed, the Celtic Goddess of Healing," ClaudiaMerrill.com, accessed January 8, 2021, https://www.claudiamerrill.com/blog/the-irish-goddess-airmed.

Apollo (Greek): Apollo is a major figure in the Olympic pantheon, and has many associations, including prophecy, oracles, music, poetry, archery, medicine, and healing. A solar deity, his symbolism includes the lyre and the laurel wreath, which signifies knowledge and academic excellence. Apollo had the power to cause or cure deadly diseases and plague. His association with medicine is so deep, the Hippocratic Oath (a version of which modern doctors still swear) begins with, "I swear by Apollo the physician." In Greek mythology, Apollo is considered to be the original source of health and healing, and the father of the mortal Asclepius, the Greek god of medicine. If drawing from the original source of healing power appeals to you, you might ask for Apollo's presence in your Sacred Massage sessions.

Asclepius/Asklepios (Greek): When discussing the god of medicine, Asclepius is often the first name to arise. His lore is so substantial that his symbol of a snake winding around its staff—the Rod of Asclepius—is still a symbol of modern medical practice. He was said to be the mortal son of the Greek god Apollo, who gave him the gift of healing and shared the secrets of medicine using plants and herbs. Asclepius' ability to heal was so powerful, he was able to raise the dead, for which he was punished by Zeus, who was outraged by his impiety.[31] Along with Apollo, Asclepius is included in the original Hippocratic Oath, along with his daughters, Hygieia and Panacea, each also gifted with healing energy, and who also appear in the oath. If your loved one is in need of a little medical miracle, in addition to your own Soothing Touch, you might be reinforced by Asclepius' participation.

Avolokiteshvara/Avalokitesvara (Buddhist): Avolokiteshvara is a bodhisattva of infinite compassion and mercy. A "bodhisattva" is one who has attained the ability to reach Nirvana, but out of compassion to humanity, chooses to postpone that next spiritual step in order to relieve suffering. Avolokiteshvara is a major deity in Buddhism, with multiple manifestations. In one of his images, he is said to have a thousand hands and eyes to help him see and help those who are suffering. There is speculation that Kuan Yin is one and the same with Avolokiteshvara, and that his Buddhist lore was later transformed to a female deity—Kuan Yin—in Chinese culture. Kuan Yin's mantra, "Om Mane Padmi Hum," is originally attributed to Avolokiteshvara, and later associated with Kuan Yin. The direct translation is "The jewel is in the lotus," and the mantra is chanted to transform and purify oneself

---

31. Mark Cartwright, "Asclepius," WorldHistory.org, last updated June 20, 2013, https://www.worldhistory .org/Asclepius/.

into the mindset of the Buddha. One of Avolokiteshvara's manifestations, Padma-pani, focuses upon helping those in dire need, possibly those facing a terminal condition or illness. He is believed to shorten the path of deliverance from suffering.[32] If compassion and mercy are at the core of your massage intentions, you might include Avolokiteshvara. If your loved one is suffering with extreme pain or illness, or even end-of-life issues, Padmapani may provide support and minimize suffering.

Brigid (Celtic): Brigid is amongst the Great Mother Goddesses. She is multitalented and multifaceted, and often described or depicted as having fiery red hair and standing at a forge doing ironwork. This was no shrinking violet. Forging takes mighty strength and endurance, and Brigid is one mighty goddess. In addition to forging and fire, her associations include poetry, protection of animals (particularly farm animals, and of those, especially sheep), and sacred wells and rivers in Ireland, Wales, and England. She is also a goddess of purification and healing, particularly healing waters. The Pagan sabbat called "Imbolc" (known as "Candlemas" in Christian traditions) falls on or near February second and is traditionally dedicated to honoring Brigid. She is also known as Bhride, Brigit, Brig, Britta, Brigantia, and Saint Brigid. If your Sacred Massage goal is to provide healing and wash away illness, pain, or stress, and to return to strength and vitality, Brigid is a powerful divine ally.

Changing Woman (Dineh/Navajo): This creation goddess of the Dineh (Navajo) people has a story rich with lore, amongst which is her ability for self-renewal.[33] Whenever her age began to show, she would walk to the west until she found her younger self, which restored her youth. This story is considered to be an allegory of the perpetually changing seasons, from spring to winter. Changing Woman is associated with the sun, sheep, corn, the earth, and the seasons, and is beloved and honored as benevolent and nurturing. She is also known as Asdzáá Nádleehé and Estsánatlehi. If rejuvenation and restoration is your Sacred Massage goal, Changing Woman could be your inspirational deity.

Eir (Norse): Her name means "help" or "mercy," and although one of the Valkyries, who are associated with battle and death, Eir chose amongst the injured on the battlefield which would live and recover. She is associated with healing lore and

---

32. Eva Rudy Jansen, *The Book of Buddhas: Ritual Symbolism used on Buddhist Statuary and Ritual Objects* (Holland: Binkey Kok Publications, 2006), 57.

33. Patricia Monaghan, *Encyclopedia of Goddesses & Heroines* (Novato, CA: New World Library, 2014), 319; Twin Rocks Trading Post, "Navajo Changing Woman," Twinrocks.com, accessed July 16, 2022, https://twinrocks.com/legends/dieties/navajo-changing-woman.html.

with copper, which was used in healing ceremonies. She is venerated as "the pre-eminent and principal healer" in Norse tradition.[34] Before males dominated the medical field, women were considered the main healers in many ancient cultures. Amongst Eir's associations are mortars and pestles, healing instruments, bandages, saunas, healing herbs, home remedies, and folk medicine. If your Sacred Massage goal is healing following a debilitating illness, injury or surgery, you might include Eir in your work.

Hippocrates (Greek): Although he was a mortal human being, a discussion of healing energy wouldn't be complete without mention of Hippocrates, declared by many as "The Father of Medicine." Inspired by the lore of Asclepius, Hippocrates stepped away from the notion that healing was the work of the gods, and believed that illnesses had natural causes and should be separated from religious rituals.[35] Hippocrates promoted a wholistic approach to health and healing, including the importance of diet, exercise, and rest. He also created the "humoral theory," which proposes that health comes from the balance of the humors of the human body: blood, phlegm, yellow bile, and black bile. Hippocrates insisted upon a high ethical standard for practicing medicine, and the original oath for physicians, the Hippocratic Oath, bears his name. Amongst the most well-known phrases from this oath is "do no harm." If you are struggling with the notion of including deity in your Sacred Massage practice, you might find spiritual inspiration by honoring Hippocrates in your work. Artwork and statuary bearing his image are easily found should you wish to create your own altar to honor him.

Hygieia (Greek): This goddess of health was the daughter of Asclepius. Both are honored as protective deities, and were sometimes worshipped together. In addition to both physical and mental health, Hygieia is also associated with cleanliness and sanitation, and is usually shown holding a bowl of milk, from which she feeds a snake or serpent. Asclepius is also associated with a snake, which is wrapped around his staff. Hygieia's name is the root for the word "hygiene." In ancient times, it was believed that invoking Hygieia could prevent illness or restore health from an illness without lingering issues. She is amongst the deities invoked in the original

---

34. Ydalir, "Norse Gods: Eir," Ydalir.ca, accessed February 25, 2022, http://ydalir.ca/norsegods/eir/.

35. Ingenia, "Hippocrates: The Ultimate Greek Healer," IngeniaHistory.com, accessed February 27, 2021, https://www.ingeniahistory.com/post/hippocrates-greek-medicine.

Hippocratic Oath.[36] If health, wellness, purifying, healing, and recovery are your Sacred Massage goals, Hygieia might provide guidance. In Roman mythology, the counterpart to Hygieia is the goddess Sirona, with essentially the same lineage and attributes, but with additional connotations and symbology. Sirona's main attribute, however, is still healing.[37]

Jesus (Christian): Although Jesus was an actual human, and therefore technically not a god, Christians believe he is the son of God, an aspect of God, or God himself. Rather than tangle over these perspectives, we'll focus on how Jesus might be a wonderful Sacred Massage deity. Many of Jesus' stories surround his power to heal through touch, and also spotlight his compassion and insight. The Christian ritual of "laying on of hands" for healing, blessing, and various religious services originates with Jesus and his divine ability to cure with his touch. He is venerated for healing the sick, and Bible stories tell that merely touching his clothing could provide healing. Jesus healed leprosy with his touch, during a time when people with this disease were ostracized. No one would come near them, let alone touch them. Jesus placed compassion above prejudice. Finding symbolism for Jesus is simple; the Christian cross is ubiquitous. However, there are other symbols associated with Jesus that focus more upon healing, hope, and love, such as a dove or lamb, or divinely empowered hands. Images of Jesus are abundant and easily found. If you feel drawn to healing through touch, particularly if your loved one has a condition or illness that others fear or avoid, Jesus could inspire fearless, loving devotion, compassion, and mercy—even if you aren't Christian. (Here's a fun fact—Jesus wasn't either.)

Isis/Aset (Egyptian): Although the Egyptian deities Thoth and Sekhmet are also considered to be healing deities alongside Isis, for our purposes, the Great Mother Goddess Isis is the best fit. Like several other deities mentioned, Isis has many associations, including fertility, motherhood, healing, protection, and magic. She is amongst the most prominent of the Egyptian deities, known worldwide. Isis' healing powers were so extraordinary, she was able to bring the Egyptian god Osiris back from the dead. She is often depicted with magnificent, colorful wings, which she spreads out from her body, and usually wearing a headdress of a solar disk and

---

36. Mike Greenberg, "Who Was the Goddess Hygieia?" Mythology Source, accessed April 26, 2021, https://mythologysource.com/goddess-hygieia/.

37. Atlantic Religion, "Sirona—Another Syncretic Guise of the Celtic 'Great Goddess'," The Atlantic Religion, last updated August 29, 2014, https://atlanticreligion.com/2014/08/29/sirona-another-syncretic-guise-of-the-celtic-great-goddess/.

cow's horns. Amongst her symbols are wings and the "tyet," also called the Knot of Isis or Girdle of Isis, which bears resemblance to the ankh, symbolizing eternal life. If you seek the power of a Great Mother Goddess, who spans both deity and magical ability, the protective wings of Isis may lift you.

Krishna (Hindu): Lord Krishna is one of the avatars (representations) of Vishnu, one of the principal Hindu deities. This beloved deity is associated with many qualities, including music, dance, flutes, joy, love, beauty, and bliss, and is considered to be the savior of humanity and the remover of all suffering. Krishna is usually depicted with blue skin and colorful silk clothing, and adorned with a golden jeweled crown and ornate jewelry. He is often holding a flute and sometimes in a dancing posture with one leg bent in front of the other. He is associated with peacocks and cows, which are sacred to Indian people. Even though the stories of Krishna stretch back to antiquity, he is to this day the most popular of Hindu divinities.[38] If one of your massage goals is to remove suffering (whether physical or mental), and bring joy and bliss into your Sacred Massage, find out more about Krishna.

Kuan Yin (Buddhist/Chinese): Like Avalokiteshvara, Kuan Yin was a "bodhisattva." In her book *Kuan Yin—Accessing the Power of the Divine Feminine*, Daniela Schenker explains that Kuan Yin's lore parallels Avalokiteshvara's, and may actually have been repurposed from his.[39] She also postponed entering Nirvana, choosing instead to stay back and devote herself to relieving suffering. Schenker says that as Kuan Yin "stood at the verge of this final threshold in contemplation, she heard shouts and cries of suffering emanating from all sentient beings, spreading about her like a great wave. So profoundly was she moved by the pain of the world's beings that her heart began to shake, and she knew that she could not yet leave the world behind."[40] Kuan Yin devotes herself to easing suffering, putting this ahead of her own needs and desires.

The symbols associated with Kuan Yin include the lotus and a small slender vase from which she pours wisdom and compassion out over humanity. Amongst the fascinating stories of Kuan Yin is her relationship to the peacock, which was once a plain, brown bird. Displeased with humanity's bickering and fighting, she passed

---

38. Temple Purhoit, "Lord Krishna—Hindu Gods and Deities," TemplePurhoit.org, accessed February 25, 2022. https://www.templepurohit.com/hindu-gods-and-deities/lord-krishna/.

39. Daniela Schenker, *Kuan Yin: Accessing the Power of the Divine Feminine* (Boulder, CO: Sounds True, 2007), 13–19.

40. Schenker, *Kuan Yin: Accessing the Power of the Divine Feminine*, 1.

her hands over the bird, transforming the plain feathers to luminous colors. At the end of each grand tail feather, she placed an eye, through which the peacock would watch over humanity and report any transgressions back to Kuan Yin. When we notice a peacock, it's a sign that "Kuan Yin is compassionately watching over us."[41] Kuan Yin's is also known as Guanyin, Guan Yin, Quan Yin, and Kwan Yin.

If a heart filled with peaceful, pure compassion resonates with you, invite Kuan Yin into your heart and your massage sessions.

Mary/Virgin Mary (Catholic, Christian): Like Jesus, the Virgin Mary (also called Holy Mother, Blessed Mother, and Our Lady) also existed in human form. However, since her humble beginnings as the mother of Jesus Christ in a cold, stark stable in Bethlehem, Mary has become a central figure in her own right, and a source of comfort and adoration amongst Christians, most notably Catholics. Mary is associated with maternal love, compassion, and faith, and an entity many people turn to, and pray to, in times of uncertainty and need. She might be an appropriate dedication figure for you if you prefer to stick with a Christian/Catholic pantheon and/or if your loved one is a devoted Catholic. Part of your Sacred Massage session might even include prayers to the Virgin Mother, and images of her are easily found in artwork, statues, and jewelry.

Panacea (Greek): Like Hygieia, the goddess Panacea (Panakeia) is amongst the deities invoked in the original Hippocratic Oath. She is a daughter of Asclepius and sister of Hygieia, and is associated with cures. Her name means "all-healing," and is a common word in the English language, meaning "a solution or remedy for all difficulties or diseases." Her particular curing power is creating poultices or potions to promote healing and and recovery from sickness. If you are interested in creating your own homemade oils, lotions, or balms to use in your Sacred Massage, you might invoke the goddess Panacea as you create them. You don't need to have fancy massage oils to do massage. You can create your own oils and lotions at home from a variety of common items, such as olive, sesame, or coconut oil, shea butter, and beeswax, and infuse them with the divine energy of your choice.

Selene (Greek): In Greek mythology, Selene wasn't merely the goddess of the moon, she *was* the moon. If you've ever stood outside under a full moon, you may have simultaneously experienced a divine energy and also an incredible peacefulness. The full moon is iconic in most every culture and the one thing seen by every

41. Schenker, *Kuan Yin: Accessing the Power of the Divine Feminine*, 131–132.

human since the dawn of time. Selene's power is inducing sleep and illuminating the night.[42] If your loved one struggles with anxiety, insomnia, or night terrors, Selene may serve as a perfect divine inspiration for calming and quieting these issues. The translucent white crystal called "Selenite" is named after this goddess of calm and rest. Selene is known as "Luna" in Roman mythology. She is sometimes depicted as driving a horse-drawn chariot across the night sky, while wearing a crescent moon-shaped headdress.

Tara (Buddhism/Tibetan, Hinduism): Many aspects of Tara's lore correlate to those of Kuan Yin, and some theorize that Kuan Yin's mythology is actually a version of Tara's. Tara's legend springs from Avolokiteshvara, who became so overwhelmed with his task of easing humanity's suffering that two tears fell from his eyes, one becoming White Tara, and the other, Green Tara.[43] In both Buddhism and Hinduism, Tara liberates humans and souls from suffering, and is an avatar of the Great Mother Goddess in Hinduism, Mahadevi. Tara is also a Great Mother Goddess herself, and the Mother of all Buddhas in Buddhism, sometimes called "Mother Tara."[44] Like Kuan Yin, Tara also has a mantra: "Om Tare Tuttare Ture Svaha," which praises Tara and requests her assistance, and is chanted in Buddhist practices. Tara has twenty-one forms, each with particular attributes. Some of her most popular forms are named by color—Green Tara, White Tara, Blue Tara, Red Tara, etc. For massage, White Tara is a perfect fit. She has eyes on her palms and feet, as well as a third eye on her forehead, which symbolize her attentiveness to humanity. She sometimes holds a white lotus blossom, signifying purity. White Tara embodies compassion, and is invoked for physical, spiritual, and psychological healing. White Tara is specifically associated with longevity.[45] If you seek a watchful goddess that inspires healing and longevity, White Tara may be the deity you're looking for.

Yemaya (Yoruba): Yemaya is an Orisha (a Yoruban deity), springing from the spiritual lore of Nigeria. Another of the Great Mother Goddesses, she is known as the ocean goddess of creation. She is associated with home, fertility, life and protection of

---

42. deTraci Regula, "Selene, Greek Goddess of the Moon," ThoughtCo, last updated June 26, 2019, https://www.thoughtco.com/greek-mythology-selene-1526204.

43. Schenker, *Kuan Yin: Accessing the Power of the Divine Feminine*, 25.

44. Mindy Newman, "Embodying the Healing Mother," Tricycle: The Buddhist Review, accessed February 26, 2022, https://tricycle.org/magazine/mother-tara-practice/.

45. Joshua Mark, "Tara," World History Encyclopedia, accessed August 9, 2021, https://www.worldhistory.org/Tara_(Goddess)/.

life, childbirth, love, change, comfort, and inspiration, and also with water, particularly the surface of the ocean and rivers. In the Yoruba creation myth, she chose to end her life as she was giving birth. Her waters broke, causing the great flood that inundated the world and the Seven Seas. The first humans, Obafalom and Lyaa, formed from her bones, and became the ancestors of all humanity.[46] Yemaya's lore was carried to other lands on slave ships, serving as a source of comfort and protection to those kidnapped and imprisoned in their holds, and as they arrived on foreign shores and were held as slaves. Yemaya is a source of motherly protection and comfort, and might calm a loved one who is undergoing turbulent challenges, situations, emotions, and thoughts, or situations out of their control. Yemaya is sometimes equated with the Virgin Mary, and her other names include Yemoja and Yemanga. Her symbols include pearls, conch shells, cowrie shells, ileke beads, the number 7 (for the seven seas), and the colors blue, white, and silver.

Angels

Angels, although divine, are not deities. Many of us imagine angels in relation to the religion we practice or grew up with, or common angel imagery, which is everywhere. Although we often refer to angels as "he" or "she," angels are neither male or female. Gender is a human characteristic, not an angelic one. While there are stories of angels presenting themselves in winged human form, I suspect that's mainly because we would be utterly overwhelmed by their pure energetic form. A human form is easier for us to wrap our relatively small minds around.

My own inspiration for including angels in spiritual practices comes from Silver RavenWolf's book *Angels: Companions in Magick*. I was captivated by angelic energy right in the introduction: "… angels appear to transcend all cultures, races, and systems. Angels are part of human history and civilization … They don't belong to any one particular religion … In truth, these religions only support the existence of angels, they didn't create them." A particular line from Silver's introduction just rings like a bell: "To call on an angel is to rise above religious dogma and touch the universal spirit."[47]

Silver's book is a comprehensive exploration of the angelic realm, how to interact with it, and how to incorporate it into magical work. It includes a thorough explanation

---

46. Goddess Gift, "Yemaya: Goddess of the Ocean and of the New Year," Goddess Gift, accessed February 25, 2022, https://www.goddessgift.com/goddess-info/meet-the-goddesses/yemaya/yemaya-unabridged/.

47. Silver RavenWolf, *Angels: Companions in Magick* (Woodbury, MN: Llewellyn Publications, 2019), x.

of the various angelic realms and entities, including seraphim, cherubim, archangels, and angels/guardian angels.[48]

Seraphim are associated with the divine Spirit (or God) itself, and are described as "pure love, light, and fire." There are four "chief" angels, corresponding to the four earthly winds—north, east, west, and south. Amongst their core purposes is to "encircle divinity to ensure its continued existence and funnel that energy toward us so we can keep going." Seraphim are typically called upon for big-ticket concerns, such as humanitarian or planetary causes, and are immensely powerful and possibly fearsome for humanity to behold.

Cherubim "function as the guardians of light and stars." They also create and channel positive energy. However, they aren't the chubby winged babies that are the darlings of the art world and our most familiar angelic image. They're much more powerful than that and far less adorable, and include some of the mighty archangels. Cherubim are called upon for protection, wisdom, and knowledge.

Archangels are crossovers of the seraphim and cherubim realms. Some believe it unwise or even dangerous to address archangels by name, and instead refer to them by the winds, directions, or energies with which they are associated.[49]

- Ariel (north), the guardian of visions, dreams, and prophecy; protector of psychics, journalists, teachers, and writers; overseeing the work of all nature spirits; in charge of natural phenomena such as tornadoes, hurricanes, thunderstorms, volcanoes, and earthquakes. This cherub sometimes assists Raphael in healing humanity.
- Raphael (east) is the "shining healer," and oversees sickness and disease. He heals through "love, joy, light, prayer, compassion, and honor," and is the "patron angel of doctors, nurses, midwives, alternative healers, travelers, and those who have lost their sight." He is also an angel of laughter and humor, and amongst the cherubim.
- Michael (south) is an avenging angel and amongst the seraphim. He is prominent in several fundamental religions, sometimes carrying a flaming or glowing sword. Silver describes him as the "Terminator of the angelic realms."[50] He is a guardian of law enforcement and armed forces personnel, and is a brave and fierce protector.

---

48. RavenWolf, *Angels: Companions in Magick*, 43–52.

49. RavenWolf, *Angels: Companions in Magick*, 22–34.

50. RavenWolf, *Angels: Companions in Magick*, 26.

- Gabriel (west) is a cherub of resurrection, transformation, and mystery, as well as the opposing energies of birth and death, and mercy and vengeance. She governs paradise and the moon, guards goddess energy on earth, and is associated with flowers and beauty, as well as winged white horses.

Angels/Guardian Angels are our go-to angels. They have relationships with humanity, and may be focused upon one particular person. They "funnel energies from us to the divine, and from the divine down to us," says Silver. They may even follow us through all of our earthly incarnations, from lifetime to lifetime. They defend us and assist us, but with a catch: They can't help us unless we ask them to. Silver advises, "When asking the angels for assistance, be sure to keep your heart and mind pure, and ask that the best solution for everyone manifest, or that you be treated in a fair and thoughtful manner."[51]

There is a universe of divine angelic energy to explore in your search for the angel that meets your Sacred Massage intentions, and a vast array of angelic images to draw upon if you wish to include an altar or visual prompts in your massage space or meditation. A basic starting point with angels might be to connect with your own guardian angel, while also recognizing that this divine entity may not be human-like, but experienced as energy, synchronicities, feelings, thoughts, or dreams. Experiencing angelic communication is a truly mind-opening experience. Begin simply by inviting your guardian angel into your life. Although you can do all sorts of research in all sorts of places, an angelic relationship forms by *doing*. I learned this firsthand while following Silver's recommendations for communicating with my guardian angel while doing research for this book. Prior to that, I didn't really view angels as in my wheelhouse. However, after feeling the skepticism and trying it anyway, I feel entirely differently about angels now. I know what I experienced, and it revealed to me that they're there—and that includes my own. Guardian angels? Absolutely *yes*.

Incorporating the Divine into Your Life

We've touched but a tiny fraction of the diverse divine universe, and hopefully I've sparked your curiosity to start exploring and discovering the deity or deities you most resonate with. You can google "healing deities" or "healing gods/goddesses," combined with your own culture, religion, nationality, or simple curiosity, such as "Tahitian healing deities" or "African goddess of compassion." If you can google it, you can find it. There's a myriad of books and information on deities, and angels too.

---

51. RavenWolf, *Angels: Companions in Magick*, 40.

While exploring these deities, particularly those associated with religions still practiced today, be aware that many are sacred to vast numbers of people. When you invite a deity into your life, do so with respect not only to that deity, but also to any culture or religion with which it's associated. Remember our earlier discussion about cultural appropriation. This applies to religions and their associated deities too. Just because you adore Lakshmi, for example, doesn't make you Hindu. That said, if you feel a deep pull toward a deity, your relationship with that deity can be strengthened by striving to live and behave in such a way that doesn't offend or conflict with that deity and its associated religious beliefs and practices. If you want to align with Lakshmi, you might want to rethink your love of a juicy T-bone steak. Remember, many of these religions are practiced by millions of people worldwide, and although the beliefs are ancient, the religion is still alive, and cherished and practiced today. Treat those religions with the respect they deserve.

Searching for the Divine with a pure, open, curious heart will lead you to fascinating discoveries, and legions of deities you never heard of before. Some may jump out to you as if to say, "Me! Pick me!" Don't blow that off. Intuition and serendipity are the roots of magic, which we'll explore in the next chapter. If you're drawn to a deity, even if you don't understand why, go with it. See what that deity has to offer. When Spirit taps your shoulder…pay attention!

Really get to know that deity, rather than limiting your relationship to massage sessions. Involve it in your life, and honor it. Keep studying and finding out more. Create altars to honor your deity, and adorn them with beautiful and meaningful items, like flowers, incense, candles, and symbols associated with that deity. When that deity really means something to you, it will be that much more fulfilling for your massage sessions.

Above all, don't approach your deity only when you need or want something. Deities aren't Alexa or Siri, sitting there silently waiting for you to ask them for something. Unlike Alexa or Siri, if you ignore your deity until you want something, that deity might start ignoring you back. We all know someone who only calls when they want something, and isn't that person a drag? Don't be "that person" with your deity. A relationship with a deity is an ongoing, growing, blossoming, living process. It's like any good relationship—they don't just happen, they require nurturing, attention, and effort.

Chapter 5

Let's Make Magic

Infusing your massage session with magical intention creates the tone and framework for Sacred Massage, and sets it apart from a regular massage, which is focused mainly on relaxation and relieving tension and minor aches and pains. There's huge value in plain old massage, but Sacred Massage takes it "next level."

Just like our exploration of deity, there's a dizzying number of ways to do magic, many of which are a part of Pagan traditions. The numbers of ways to perform a ritual or do magic would be impossible to calculate. Many practices have certain basic practices in common, but there's also a lot of diversity. There's no "right" way to do magic or ritual—each person or group creates their own version of ritual or magical practice. For our Sacred Massage purposes, we're not going to do any elaborate ceremonial magic. We'll focus on simple magical approaches that lend themselves to healing, relaxation, and the channeling of divine love and compassion. We'll also explore ways for you to magically boost your confidence and focus before beginning your massage session. We'll learn a basic magical ritual, and later on, use it as a template for creating a Sacred Massage ritual.

What Is Magic?

When you think of magic, do you imagine a mysterious cape-clad figure tapping a wand on an empty box, releasing a flock of doves? Or a cackling green cartoon witch with warts and ratty hair transforming someone into a toad? A genie creating a pile of gold at your feet with a nod of his magical, mystical head? Or maybe a teenage witch movie where marginalized girls with too much black eyeliner get revenge on those who mistreated them by summoning hurricanes and lightning? These are all quite familiar and entertaining, but that's really all they are: entertaining.

In the Pagan community, "magic" is frequently spelled with a "k" at the end, to differentiate it from sideshow "Watch me pull a rabbit out of my hat" hocus pocus. As opposed to fun, fantasy, and entertainment, Pagan magic is a process designed to result in, or manifest, a specific goal. One is just for fun; the other is done for a specific reason and specific result.

Distilled to its simplest form, magic has three parts: intention, implementation, and manifestation. Intention is the specific goal you want. Implementation is the things you do to make that goal happen. Manifestation is releasing your intention to the universe to let it fulfill your goal.

Studying magic is a perpetual learning process that requires practice and study, just like woodworking or playing the piano. That's the "craftsmanship" component of magic—the implementation. But there's also the metaphysical side of magic, when the implementation results in manifestation. How the heck does *that* work? I personally think it's all about vibration. Everything within the universe vibrates, from the heavenly bodies out across the cosmos to the space between the sub-atomic particles within your own cells.[52] In between all those vibrating objects, whether a planet or a molecule in your body, is a sea of dark matter and dark energy. Scientists don't really know what it is or what it does, but they know it's there.

Quantum mechanics experiments have proven that an action in one place can affect an action in another, even in the absence of physical contact. This has been demonstrated by experiments on simple particles, and how they behave in different situations.[53] They don't know *why* this occurs, only *that* it occurs. My own theory is that one day, they'll discover that vibration is the reason, and that vibration ripples through that sea of dark matter and dark energy, like a vast pond. If you wiggle your fingers in the water, it makes little ripples outward. At some point, your eye can't see the ripples, but the particles in the water are still moving. I believe that we set a magical vibration in motion, and push it out to the universe, where that vibration is received and responded to.

Does magic always work? Nope. But there are reasons for that, from simple user error to the universe in its infinite wisdom recognizing that what you asked for would be disastrous. Sort of like if your seven-year-old really, really wants a chainsaw. That can only turn out badly. The answer is no. That's why when I do magical work, whatever my intention, I

---

52. The Conversation, "Could Consciousness All Come Down to the Way Things Vibrate?", last updated November 9, 2018, https://theconversation.com/could-consciousness-all-come-down-to-the-way-things-vibrate-103070.

53. Weizmann Institute of Science, "Quantum Theory Demonstrated: Observation Affects Reality," Science Daily, February 26, 1998, https://www.sciencedaily.com/releases/1998/02/980227055013.htm.

always add, "with harm to none and for the greater good of all." When the universe gives me a "no," I assume there were unforeseen negative consequences or harm that would have resulted from my magical petition.

While many mock and ridicule magic, there was once a time when people of limited imagination, intellect, and information mocked and ridiculed anyone who disputed that the earth was flat, and also the center of the universe. Our understanding of the earth and the cosmos was so limited, and our arrogance so immense, that popular belief at that time was mostly egocentric fantasy. I believe that one day, scientists will discover what magical practitioners have always known: Magic exists. They may discover that magic and science are two sides of the same metaphysical coin. And I predict that, when they accomplish this, it will be within the field of quantum mechanics. Until then, to those who declare "You have no proof that magic exists," I reply, "Absence of evidence is not evidence of absence." And also, "Temper your arrogance with an awareness of your limited imagination, intellect, and information."

Within our Sacred Massage practice, we're not going to get lost in the high weeds of whether or not magic exists or works. We're going to take it as a given that it does, and proceed from there. Just keep an open mind, be open to possibility, and see for yourself if it makes a difference in both your internal and external experience. Set your skepticism aside for our time together. If you want it back when we're finished, it will be right where you left it.

As we explore the magical realm, bear in mind that magic is sometimes a whisper, not a shout. You must be still enough to hear the magical whispers amid life's cacophony. Also, manifestations don't always materialize in the form you expected. For example, if your magical intention is a new job, that could be manifested as a promotion *or* a layoff. That's why you must be specific when crafting your intention. Don't leave it up to the universe to interpret your message. The universe can be very creative in its responses!

Chances are, you've already done magic and didn't know it. Have you ever made some soup for a loved one who wasn't feeling well, wishing for their recovery as you cooked, maybe adding a special spice or herb, and then serving it to that person with the most loving intentions and then … they felt better? Well, congratulations—you've done kitchen magic. Let's find out how magic works in massage.

The Magical Environment

The first step of massage magic is to deciding where you'll do it. The area should be as quiet and undisturbed as possible. Make the area special, just as you would spiff up your living room if you were expecting guests, or decorate for a special party. It's amazing how things as simple as lowering the lights, burning a candle, and playing relaxing massage music can transform a room into a place for relaxation, trust, and healing. You can do a little magical preparation on yourself too. It's like dressing up for that special party. You really do feel and behave differently in your favorite party dress or suit than if you showed up in your PJ pants and bunny slippers, with your hair looking like a bird just picked through it for nesting material. An external change can prompt internal change.

Creating a magical environment isn't absolutely necessary to do magical work, and you may have no option other than to do your massage session in someone else's space, or even a public space like a nursing home or hospital. But if you do have the option to make your massage space magical, it will really enhance the experience.

Working From Home

Before starting your massage magic, choose a space for your sessions. The optimal situation is a space dedicated to massage exclusively. If you don't have that luxury, find a spot in your home where you could do massage as privately and peacefully as possible. It might not be perfect, but just do your best, even if that means working out of your living room. (Which I have done before, when I still had kids in the house!) Even if your massage space serves dual purposes, you can still use some of the ideas in this chapter to make shared spaces a little more magical while you work.

Your Special Sacred Spot

When you've chosen your Sacred Massage spot, look at it with fresh eyes. Are there things there that aren't conducive to relaxation? Move or cover these things when you massage, and do your best to create a peaceful, relaxing tone. My massage office is also my writing office, as well as my magical workspace. That's a lot of stuff for a small room. However, there aren't any items in the room that distract from a relaxed mood. Anything that's less than optimal for a magical, massage-y mood has been hidden in wicker baskets that slide into a bookcase. All the colors in the room are calming pastels—lavender, grey, beige, white, and baby blue. The room is adorned with many of my magical items, such as crystals, candles, seashells, and goddess figurines. Some might think they're just decorations, but no, they're all magically significant.

If you'll also be working in a room that serves dual, or triple, services, look around—does anything catch your eye that creates anxiety or sadness, or just generates too much energy? If so, move these things elsewhere while you're working, or cover them up with a cloth in a soft color. When creating a certain tone, removing things can be more important than adding things. Avoid bright, saturated colors unless your intention is to lift and revive your loved one's energy. Bright colors wake you up and soft pastels calm you down.

If there's a lot of clutter (clutter clogs and bogs down the flow of energy or "chi"), get some pretty hat boxes or storage boxes at a home goods store, and stack them so they look more like a decoration than a storage system. You want space for both you *and* energy to move freely as you work. Your Sacred Massage venture is a great excuse for getting rid of things you don't really need, want, or use.

Activity
CLEANSING AND DEDICATING YOUR MASSAGE SPACE

When you've chosen your Sacred Massage spot and have it arranged the way you want, energetically cleansing the area transforms this space into a magical space. Before doing a magical ritual, you'd energetically cleanse the area. There are many ways to do this, but a common one is sweeping any negative or unwanted energy out the door with a real or imaginary broom.

Working with this magical sweeping concept, begin your magical cleansing at the wall opposite the doorway. Using a real broom and dustpan, or just using your hands to imitate them, sweep up all the negative or stagnant energy toward the doorway. When you reach the doorway, sweep it all into your dustpan. If the doorway leads to the outside, take the dustpan outside and fling away that oogie energetic sludge, and declare it, out loud, "Banished!" If the doorway leads to another room, carry your magical dustpan to an external door, and fling it away. If you want a little extra magical oomph, sprinkle a line of salt across the outside threshold of the door after banishing that energy. Then, slam that door shut with confidence. That negative energy is declared unwelcome, and uninvited.

After cleansing your massage space, you'll dedicate it as your own special magical massage spot. You'll need some incense, dried bay leaves, or sage, or a mister filled with magical or moon-blessed water (more on all these items in a bit) for magically clearing away any negative energy from your space, and blessing or claiming it as a safe place with only helpful, supportive energies. Starting at the north side of the room and moving clockwise, swirl the smoke or spray the mist as you think or chant a mantra, such as "Only healing … only peace …" You can use that mantra, or create one of your own.

When you're finished, have a seat in this special spot. Celebrate it by lighting a candle or playing some music. Here it is: your own sacred healing place. Notice how that feels. Do you feel a little different already? Maybe like some sacred healing energy is starting to blossom? Wonderful! Because in this space, you *are* a healer.

(*A little note about sage: White sage is sacred to indigenous people in this country, and should not be used outside that community unless you purchase from an indigenous seller or grow it yourself.)*

Working Away from Home

Creating a magical massage space in your own home is fairly simple. However, if you must go to someone else's home, or a hospital or nursing home, you'll have to be a bit more creative and flexible. When I would visit my father in a skilled nursing facility, it reeked of Pine Sol and misery. There were often people coming in and out of his room, and sometimes his roommate would be yelling uncontrollably in a fit of dementia or despair, or both. This is not an optimal massage situation, sacred or otherwise. If you'll be dealing with similar difficult and unpredictable circumstances, ask if there's a quiet, private room or patio where you could visit with your loved one for awhile—preferably a space where you can close the door. Another option is to take it outside. Take a walk or drive in the neighborhood (use a wheelchair for your loved one if necessary) and find a park or open space that offers some privacy and quiet—maybe under a shade tree or near a pond. Being outdoors, near nature, actually enhances calmness and healing. It's no accident that the color of the heart chakra is green.

If the neighborhood doesn't offer any relaxing options or if your loved one is confined to bed, don't despair. No matter what's going on around you, your touch can still transmit calm, comfort, and healing, right there amid the chaos. Make use of that meditation skill of swiping away intrusive thoughts, but this time you'll swipe away sounds and other intrusions: *Yup, that's a sound. Off you go.* When distracted, bring your focus and attention back to your hands, and your healing intention.

When you've found an acceptable place to do massage on your loved one, cleanse and dedicate that spot before beginning, just as you did for the spot in your home. Your hands become broom and dustpan to sweeping away negative energy and cast it off. If an external door isn't handy, dump it into a toilet or trash can. Repeat your cleansing mantra in your mind: "Only healing … only peace."

When doing massage in someone else's home or living situation, or in a hospital, you can't really redecorate those spots to your liking. However, magical prompts can be very mobile. They'll remind you that your magical, divine energy is always with you, and help you maintain your focus. You can wear a pendant or carry a crystal in your pocket, or create a little magical altar on a side table or shelf (more on altars in just a bit). Keep it simple—a small altar cloth, a nice crystal, and maybe a symbol of water or earth. You could also bring a small figurine of your healing deity and place it nearby. However, if your loved one is uncomfortable with an altar such as this, you could charge a flower in a little vase with the magical energy you want to include, and leave the flower as a gift. You could also skip the altar entirely if it goes against your loved one's preferences. An altar, and the items on it, are not truly necessary. Ultimately, magic is within *you*—not contained in things. The things simply reinforce your own magical focus and intention.

A really simple thing you can do to create an instant magical mood is to place or hang a short string of tiny LED fairy lights in the room, turn the lighting down, or off, and let the fairy lights provide the light. You'll feel the energy in the room settle down, and the magical energy rise. Little battery-operated light strings are light, portable, and simple to bring along when doing massage away from home.

If your loved one is receptive to it, they might like a calming crystal or small deity or angel statue to keep on their nightstand or a nearby shelf to maintain a magical presence when you're away. You can even create a little altar for them, if they're open to that. Explain that these gifts are meant to provide comfort while you're away, and to remind them that you'll be returning soon.

Magical Massage Tools and Supplies

We just covered the "where" of incorporating magic into your Sacred Massage—now we'll explore the "what": magical tools, items, and supplies. While magical items can inspire a richer, more mystical experience and mindset, they aren't actually necessary. You could do an entire magical working or ritual using nothing but your mind, hands, body, and voice to set your intention into motion, and the same applies to massage. You don't need a bunch of fancy things to do amazing healing magic: just your mind, hands, body, and voice, and maybe a little massage oil. That said, magical things energetically lubricate your own mind and energy, and help you focus. This is particularly helpful on days when you're sad, tired, or distracted, and need some extra support. Using magical tools and items whenever you wish, or just because you like them, certainly won't hurt anything, but to be clear: it's *you*—not the things—that creates magic.

Your Magical Massage Table

Your biggest magical massage tool is your table. It is your magical "working" altar, where you'll do your magical work—the magic happens under your hands. Although I just said that magical tools aren't really necessary for massage, a massage table is the exception— it will make a huge difference in your overall massage experience because you and your loved one will be much more comfortable.

Let's start viewing your massage table as more than merely a massage tool—let's prepare and treat it like the magical altar that it is.

Manifest That Table

A massage table isn't a luxury—it's a necessary tool. If you still haven't been able to acquire a table by the usual means or if expense is an issue, put your need out to the universe: Do a magical ritual (see section on ritual in the next chapter) with the intention of acquiring a free or very affordable massage table. They really are out there. You just need to magically attract one to you. Get that manifestation moving!

Activity

CLEANSING AND DEDICATING
YOUR MAGICAL MASSAGE TABLE

To prepare your massage table (or other work surface) for doing magical work, we'll treat it as any other magical tool and welcome it into your massage work by magically cleansing and dedicating it, just as we did with your workspace. You'll need some moon-blessed or magical water in a mister, or some incense, bay leaves, or sage, something to burn them in or on, and matches. Light the incense, bay leaves, or sage, and swirl and trail the smoke all over your table as you chant a dedication mantra, such as "Only healing … only peace." If using a mister, same thing—chant as you mist. Place your hands on your table, draw in divine love and compassion from the universe, channel it through your heart and out your hands. Trace a meaningful symbol on the table with your finger, and welcome this table into your magical practice.

More Magical Massage Tools

There are about ten gazillion tools, items, and supplies, and about twice as many ways to use them magically. You can find entire books just on crystals or candles. In this section, we'll whittle that number down to some simple items that lend themselves to massage. Think of this section like a magical smorgasbord—pick what you like and leave the rest. You can use one, some, all, or even none of these items, as you please—on an altar to attract the energies you desire for doing massage, to focus your mind for magical work or massage, or to enhance the magical energy in your massage space and keep that magical energy flowing.

Candles

Candles are probably the most universally familiar item for spiritual and magical purposes, and even just for plain old mood lighting. There's nothing like candlelight to soften the energy in a room. One way to do candle magic is to infuse the candle with your intention by speaking or breathing your intention into it, such as: "I will channel the comforting love of Yemaya to my sister." You can also scratch your intention into it with a pin or tack, maybe summarizing your intention with a few words: "healing, comfort, compassion." Place the candle in a special spot where it can't be knocked over or start a fire, and light it. Imagine as it burns that the light is emanating your intention throughout the room and your massage session, as the burning wick carries your intention to the universe for manifestation. When the candle has burned all the way down, your intention is on its way.

While scented candles are lovely, some people are very sensitive to even the faintest scents. If your loved one is amongst them, an unscented candle is best, and preferably made from soy or beeswax, because they produce little or no smoke. Anytime you can see or smell smoke, it's releasing particulate matter into the air, and that air is going into your lungs. If your loved one has asthma or allergies, that might trigger some discomfort. It's long been perceived as a "given" that wax candles are harmful; however, it turns out that the wicks with lead cores were the real culprits.[54] Lead wicks were outlawed in the United States in 2003, but to be really sure your candle doesn't have a lead wick, rub white paper over the unburned wick. If it leaves a gray mark like a pencil, it's not safe. That said, even with a safe wick, wax candles do produce smoke and soot, which doesn't fit into a practice devoted to health and wellness. Soy or beeswax are a better choice. Battery-operated faux candles are another option, providing an entirely smoke- and scent-free alternative.

Color

Color magic is simple, for massage and in general. All colors have magical energy and symbolism, and can be used to amplify or mute a particular energy. For massage, pastels— baby blue and pink, lavender, gentle greens and yellows, soft grays—will set a relaxing tone. If you wear bright red-and-white stripes or fluorescent yellow to your massage session, the energy of these colors is counter-productive for calm and relaxation. Avoid bright primary colors or fluorescents on your clothing and in the room because they raise energy. However (and there's always a however, isn't there), there might be situations where you actually *want* to raise energy, such as someone recovering from a severe illness or injury, or someone struggling with depression or fatigue.

You can do color magic with the clothing you wear, your massage sheets, blankets, or curtains, the paint on the walls, adding decor, or using that color on an altar. You can combine color magic and candle magic by picking a candle in the color that represents your magical massage intention. In general, when you want to lower energy, move toward the pastel end of the color scale. When you want to stimulate energy, move toward the full-saturation end.

Here are the magical associations with color:[55]

Red: Power, dominance, danger, willpower, romantic love, passion, seduction, fire energy; root chakra, the center of safety, security, stability, survival issues.
Orange: High energy, male energy, boldness, sexuality, creation, adventure, fun, celebration, fire energy; sacral chakra, the center of sexuality, pleasure, and procreation.

---

54. Sam Gutierrez, "Are Your Favorite Candles Slowly Poisoning You?" HouseBeautiful.com, last updated December 26, 2018, https://www.housebeautiful.com/lifestyle/a25656783/candles-bad-for-you/.

55. Debra DeAngelo, *Pagan Curious: A Beginner's Guide to Nature, Magic and Spirituality* (Woodbury, MN: Llewellyn Publications, 2022), 176–177.

Yellow: Intelligence, learning, knowledge, all matters of the mind, including writing and investigating; morning, new growth, new energy, rejuvenation, happiness, the sun, air energy; solar plexus chakra, the center of courage, self-confidence, and self-esteem.

Green: Abundance, wealth, growth, good luck, healing, earth energy; heart chakra, the center of love, joy, inner peace, and compassion.

Blue: Communication, emotions, creativity, peacefulness, serenity, calm, water energy; throat chakra, the center of expressing emotions and the heart's truth.

Purple: Intuition, insight, psychic abilities, mysticism, divination, water energy; third eye chakra, the center of intuition and wisdom.

White/Clear: Purity, innocence, the moon, the Goddess, the sacred or divine feminine, Spirit; crown chakra. In some traditions, the crown chakra is violet or lavender. I prefer the alternate symbology of white or a clear prism. The crown chakra is spiritual connection to the Divine. When light—regular or divine—passes through a clear prism, it emanates all the colors of the rainbow, and the chakras.

Pink: Friendship, tenderness, softness, self-love, motherly love, spiritual healing, female energy.

Hot Pink: Brightness, boldness, joy, parties, standing out in a crowd, fire energy.

Gray: Grounding, neutrality, calming, dulling, toning down, blending in.

Black: Indomitable spirit, force, power, protection, magic, the shadow, repelling, banishing, hexes, the new moon, invisibility.

Brown: Grounding, protection, safety, stability, calm, earth energy.

Neon (any color): Attracting attention; any color's magical energy brightened to full saturation.

Pastels (any color): Gentleness, toning down, lightness, delicateness, air energy.

Silver: Moon magic, the Goddess, spiritual protection, female energy, yin.

Gold: Sun magic, the God, power, money, wealth, male energy, yang.

Crystals and Stones

Crystals and stones are formed within the earth, where they are infused with the grounded, calming energy of Mother Earth. In magic, the element of earth pertains to nature and the ground, and our bodies and health. Earth is associated with north, midnight, and winter. The deep depths of winter are when many animals hibernate, sleeping and healing until spring returns. Earth is a slow, steady heartbeat, inspiring us to take all the time we need to heal.

Whatever your magical intention or need, there's a corresponding crystal or stone. You can find them online or at a rock or metaphysical shop, or you can take a walk out in nature and pick up a stone that catches your eye and infuse it with your own magical intention by writing or engraving on it, or breathing your intention into it just like a candle. Treat is as though it's just as magical as a crystal from a shop—because it is. You've charged it with your magical intention.

Use crystals to attract the particular magical energy you want, and project it into your Sacred Massage or toward your loved one. Set them in your massage area, wear them as pendants, or carry them in a little bag in your pocket.

Before using your crystals or stones, clean them with a soft cloth or brush. Some may be gently washed, but check first because water may damage certain crystals, like selenite. After cleaning the crystal or stone, magically cleanse it by passing it through smoke (incense, bay leaf, or sage) or set it under the light of the full moon for an entire night. If weather is an issue, put it in a clear jar or plastic bag. You can also place it near a window where the moonlight streams inside. After cleansing, hold the crystal in your palms, communicate to it the energy you want it to attract, and welcome it into your magical life.

There's a dizzying array of magical energies associated with crystals. Here are some crystals and stones that I find particularly harmonious for massage, relaxation, and healing:[56]

> **Agate:** Grounding, soothing, physical health and healing, survival, earth energy. Agate is a common "nothing fancy" stone—down to earth, keeping things simple and natural, and toning things down. Agates are "no drama, mama" stones. Agate brings energy down to the ground. If your loved one is habitually wound around the axle about one thing or another, agate slows and settles that energy. If your loved one is fidgety and restless, give them a smooth agate stone to tumble over in their fingers while you work, much like a worry stone.
>
> **Amethyst:** Spirituality, divine connection, calm, serenity, spiritual and emotional healing, psychic energy, third eye chakra. An all-around excellent stone for massage, meditation, and stress reduction. Amethyst supports your own efforts to understand your loved one's physical or emotional struggles. Its gentle lavender color is conducive to relaxation and calm.
>
> **Celestite:** Spiritual detox, spiritual and emotional release and healing, relaxation, stress reduction, divine connection, divine healing, angels, crown chakra, peaceful sleep.

---

56. DeAngelo, *Pagan Curious: A Beginner's Guide to Nature, Magic and Spirituality*, 177–181.

This delicate powder-blue stone is calming and particularly helpful for emotional distress or anxiety. If you've chosen angels as your massage deities, this gently calming crystal would complement that divine energy beautifully.

Charoite: Intuition, cosmic connection, divine connection, psychic energy, increased attention span, mental focus, dreams, easing fear, third eye chakra. Charoite reinforces your connection to the metaphysical plane, and gives confidence in trusting your intuition and divine guidance. It's a good choice for connecting with deities and angels. Charoite crystals with clear quartz inclusions are particularly powerful—an eye into the beyond. Like amethyst, charoite helps you to see and understand hidden struggles or pain, whether physical or psychological. Another of charoite's magical properties is to protect loved ones while they're apart. This makes charoite a perfect stone to give to a loved one who doesn't live with you, to remind them that they are safe, and that you care about them even when you're away, and that you will return. Charoite is a magical placeholder for those loved ones you can't be with all the time.

Clear Quartz: Clarity, focus, attracts divine light and energy, crown chakra, channeling energy. It can be used for any magical purpose in place of another crystal, and when placed next to another crystal, will amplify that crystal's energy. Quartz crystal is excellent for receiving messages in divination or meditation, and can be used for the same purpose in the physical world. Quartz crystals are used in radio transmission, watches, and computers, and can produce electricity when put under physical stress, such as impact or heat. Keeping a quartz crystal nearby is like having a metaphysical radio receiver on an open channel all the time. Wear a quartz pendant when you really want to tune in and understand another person's issues, or when you seek clarity, insight, and divine energy.

Fluorite: Calm, healing, stability, serenity, physical and mental health, physical and mental recovery. If lavender in color, third eye chakra. Fluorite comes in a variety of colors, most commonly translucent greens, whites, and purples, and often a combination of all three, with ribbons of each running through the stone that sometimes look like flowing water. Fluorite is very cooperative and agreeable. It will enhance the "only good vibes" energy when placed next to another crystal or stone, and it's a favorite stone for my massage office, second only to rose quartz. If you seek an all-around "let go and relax" crystal, for you or your loved one, meet your new best friend: fluorite.

Geode: Protection, Mother Earth, earth energy, hidden mysteries, intuition, psychic energy, going within, the womb. Inside their ordinary dull rock shells, geodes are tiny caves lined with crystals, often quartz or amethyst. When one's sparkling, magical inner self needs release (or conversely, needs protection), geode provides that. Geode gives comforting, protective support for those who feel broken or hopeless, or who are grieving the death of a loved one; for those whose healing will take time, and there's no immediate solution. Geodes are the crystal equivalent of holding someone in your arms for as long as need be, when quick, easy solutions aren't possible. They can curl inside geode's safe, protective cave, and hibernate there while their hearts and spirits heal, for as long as that takes. Geode is the stone of choice when there are no quick fixes; to emotional or physical trauma that only time will heal.

Jade: Money, luck, wealth, are the traditional associations with jade, but for magical massage purposes, it is also the green stone of the heart chakra, which is the source for love, compassion, and healing. Jade can balance emotions by uplifting positive energy and dissipating negative energy. Jade is easily found in jewelry and carved into figurines, and a simple jade pendant or figurine on a shelf is a simple way to include it in your massage session.

Labradorite: Intuition, the subconscious, imagination, divination, stress reduction, warding off confrontation and stress, peace, calm. This beautiful blue-gray stone with flashes of green and gold is particularly helpful when dealing with difficult people—and sometimes loved ones can be the most difficult people you know. Labradorite eases conflict and, if drama breaks out, serves as a prompt to take a step back and disengage. For example, a loved one with dementia or Autism Spectrum Disorder might become upset or agitated during a session, sometimes for no reason you can identify. Labradorite won't stop that, but it will remind you that your loved one is dealing with a situation as best they can, and that this behavior isn't "bad" or "wrong," but rather, their unique response to certain stimuli. Labradorite prompts you to be accepting rather than judgmental, while at the same time, not become swept up in the energy of the moment: *It just is what it is—no worries, we'll proceed when you're ready.* You might use labradorite when interacting with a relative or partner with whom you have a lot of emotional baggage that often triggers conflicts. Labradorite reminds you to disengage from difficult emotions, and to not take the argument bait when it's dangled in front of you.

Moonstone: The moon, the Goddess, the goddess Selene, yin, feminine energy, feminine healing and health, the female body, intuition. Moonstone eases female or menstrual issues, and enhances Goddess energy. It aligns feminine energy and the moon's. Yin energy is dark, cool, and receptive, and moonstone amplifies this internal soft but strong energy. A loved one suffering with severe menstrual cramps or endometriosis would benefit from moonstone's presence. That doesn't mean skip the doctor—it means that moonstone will be supportive in your loved one's healing journey.

Red Jasper: Family, ancestors, grounding, earth energy, root chakra. Like the root chakra, red jasper is reaffirming and reassuring when you feel unsafe. This might be a stone to wear or carry for your own emotional support, particularly when caring for a loved one facing end-of-life issues or dangerous situations. Red is the color of blood, and this stone reinforces family bonds and the bloodline of ancestors, which continue on even after separation on this physical plane. Red jasper might be an appropriate choice for a loved one who is dealing with the imminent or recent loss of a partner or relative, as a reminder that although the body may cease to be, love transcends space and time. The bloodline continues on.

Rose Quartz: Self-healing, self-love, motherly love and protection, kindness, emotional recovery, grief recovery. Nothing emits gentle, tender, healing love like rose quartz. It goes right to the heart to calm and lighten painful emotions. Rose quartz is patient, tender, and kind—a loving motherly embrace. It's perfect for healing someone else's heart, or your own, or for anyone whose self-esteem has taken a beating or for someone who drives themself so hard, they create their own physical and emotional strains. Rose quartz is my number one favorite massage stone for channeling compassion, love, and healing from my heart to someone else's. When someone needs major love and healing, I infuse a piece of rose quartz with those intentions for that person, and place it in a geode half-shell on a special healing altar. This is my little crystalline "ICU," for those who need time to nest inside and heal. I always ask someone before including them in magical work, because doing magic on someone without their permission—even with good intentions—is a magical party foul.

Tiger's-Eye: Physical strength and healing, stamina, courage, self-confidence, solar plexus chakra, fire energy. Tiger's-eye empowers you when you're feeling emotionally or physically weak or unwell. The "Eye of the Tiger" theme song from the *Rocky* movies captures tiger's eye energy, and the gold, brown, and black stripes resemble the eye of a big cat. If your loved one needs a big shot of physical strength and healing to overcome a tough health situation, particularly one that may require physical therapy, tiger's-eye will serve them well. Tiger's-eye will also invigorate you when you need extra strength or stamina to work on a loved one with particularly challenging physical issues. If you feel completely drained after working on a particular person, wear or carry tiger's-eye as a preventative measure before working on them.

Herbs, Spices, and Essential Oils

Herbs, spices, and essential oils are magical staples; however, if you plan to ingest or inhale them, or apply them to the skin, be sure to research them first because they can be highly concentrated and potent, and may require diluting first. Being ultra cautious and doing proactive research rarely hurts anyone or anything, but charging blindly ahead without the necessary information can be disastrous.

Herbs can be used magically by brewing them as tea, including them on an altar, or adding them to small magical bags or pouches to carry with you. Herbs can be infused into oil or dried and sewn into little sachets to keep under a pillow, or add natural, gentle fragrance to a massage area. You can pinch the sachets with your fingers to release more scent. You can pump up your candle magic by sprinkling or rubbing them with herbs or oils, infusing the herbs and candle with your intention. Dried herbs can be sprinkled onto a charcoal tablet as incense for magical working or ritual. I like to use essential oils to "dot" a massage space or table, which invites that oil's energy and healing properties into my massage sessions.

Another way to bring herbal magic to your massage space is to grow it in a little pot on the windowsill. Most herbs are easy to grow indoors if they have sunlight. When you grow herbs yourself, indoors or out, you infuse healing intention into them from the moment you plant them, making them extra potent for magical work. Having fresh, growing plants gives you a steady supply of magical teas or dried herbs. When using cuttings from living plants for magical work, always explain to the plant why you are cutting it, and thank it for its gift. Repay the plant by taking excellent care of it and guarding it from bugs and diseases.

Choose herbs, spices, or essential oils depending upon your magical massage intention—relaxation, healing, emotional support, etc. Over time, the scent of that herb will serve as a trigger to step into the particular mental or emotional space you desire. Most people immediately relax when they smell lavender, for example. Many of the herbs we'll be exploring can also be found in essential oils, both blends and single notes, which can be used for aromatherapy during massage to invite an emotional response—to calm and soothe, or to clear, stimulate, and brighten. Infuse the oil with your intention, just like a crystal, and then add it to your massage oil or lotion, or sprinkle it on your massage table or sheets. Some essential oils may be applied directly to the skin, but you must check the bottle first to make sure it's intended for that. Essential oils can also be used in diffusers to fill the air with their scent—and your magical intention. There are also special pendants with felt pads inside that you can drip essential oil onto and wear, to keep that magical scent moving with you all day. You can achieve the same effect by putting some oil drops on a cotton ball and stashing them in your bra between the girls, or in a shirt pocket.

As was mentioned with candles, some people are highly sensitive or even allergic to particular herbs or scents. If your loved one gets a headache, starts coughing or sneezing, has an asthma attack, or reddened eyes or skin, stop using that herb immediately and air out the room. Even if your loved one simply doesn't like the scent—don't use it. I, for example, can't stand the smell of ylang ylang, but other people just love it. No matter how much you want to infuse a session with the energies of a certain scent, if your loved one doesn't like it (or any other magical enhancement, for that matter), find another route to those energies, such as using the herbs or oils outside the massage space for your own magical reinforcement.

There are thousands of herbs, spices, and essential oils with magical or healing properties. Here are my personal favorites. These are great for massage magic because they are "crossovers"—herbs, spices, and essential oils that both the magical and medical communities agree have positive and powerful health benefits:

Basil: This favorite of all Italian chefs offers divine protection, peace, and attracting wealth. There is the familiar sweet basil we use in the kitchen, and there's also tulsi or holy basil, used in Ayurveda for calming the mind and body. Basil can easily be grown in the garden or in a pot on the windowsill. Indoors, the plant's heavenly fragrance clears and freshens the air. Sweet basil essential oil simultaneously calms and brightens the mind, but is a powerful oil that needs dilution before applying to the skin, and should not be ingested. Basil is an antioxidant, making it a natural cancer-fighter, and it may also support liver health, reduce blood sugar and inflammation, protect skin from aging, and support cardiovascular and mental health.[57]

Chamomile: Calm, soothing chamomile is particularly effective for stomach and digestive issues. The scent of pure chamomile tea immediately induces slow, deep breathing, and peace. The flower portion of the plant is most widely used. The flowers are dried for tea, but also are a lovely addition to a sachet or potpourri bag for infusing an area with peace and calm.

Clove: Clove is a warming herb that induces energy, interest, and productivity. Its heady scent could help spark energy in a loved one that is dealing with fatigue or depression. Clove essential oil may increase circulation and relieve pain, which makes it great for massage.[58] It also assists with healing, particularly skin issues. Because it's so pungent and can create a burning sensation on the skin, it's best to dilute it in a carrier oil, like sesame or olive, until you see how your loved one reacts to it. A little clove goes a long way.

Jasmine: The scent of pure bliss is jasmine. One whiff immediately elevates one's mood, and heart. Like chamomile, it's used for perfume, tea, sachets, and potpourri, but it can also be found in essential oil form. Jasmine flowers are my favorites for making moon-blessed water (instructions to follow), which has a variety of divine cleansing and blessing purposes: sprinkle it over yourself, your loved one, your massage area, or anything you'd like to bless with heavenly bliss and tranquility.

Lavender: Of all the scents associated with massage and aromatherapy, lavender towers above all others. Lavender is the go-to scent for standard massage oils and lotions, and the pure essential oil can be used directly on the skin. It has antiseptic and anti-inflammatory properties, and alleviates anxiety, insomnia, depression, and restlessness. It can even assist with fungal infections and help heal wounds.[59] The pure oil has a powerful scent, and can clear stuffy sinuses. A nice finishing touch at the end of your massage session is to put a couple drops of lavender essential oil on your fingertips, and slowly spread it in small, gentle circles over your loved one's temples. You can also dab it on your loved one's wrists or other pulse points to help

57. Yvette Brazier, "Health Benefits of Basil," MedicalNewsToday.com, last updated December 16, 2019. https://www.medicalnewstoday.com/articles/266425.

58. Meenakshi Nagdeve, "16 Surprising Benefits of Clove Oil," OrganicFacts.net, accessed June 1, 2021, https://www.organicfacts.net/health-benefits/essential-oils/health-benefits-of-clove-oil.html.

59. Joseph Nordqvist, "What are the Health Benefits and Risks of Lavender?" MedicalNewsToday.com, last updated March 4, 2019, https://www.medicalnewstoday.com/articles/265922.

induce calm before a massage, or afterwards to help them stay in their "peaceful place." If you only use one herb in your Sacred Massage, lavender would be at the top of the list. Fresh sprigs of lavender are excellent for creating your own herb-infused oil, which you can use directly on the skin or include when making lotion. One note about the pure lavender essential oil: unlike the flower itself, the essential oil is toxic, and only safe for external use.

Lemon: Smell a fresh lemon, and your mind brightens right up. It's so refreshing! Although massage is usually associated with calming and relaxing, sometimes a person needs their energy elevated, such as when dealing with depression, grief, or chronic fatigue. Lemon clears the mind when there are too many thoughts and worries bouncing off the cranial walls. It's also an energy lift for yourself when you need your mind clear and your energy ready for doing massage. Fresh lemon is simple to use—both the juice and the grated rind. You can drink it in water or tea for a fresh, bright start to the day, and offer it in water to your loved one after a massage to help clear and cleanse their digestive system, and maybe if they need to "wake up" afterwards. In a carrier oil, lemon essential oil is safe to apply to the skin, but may create sun sensitivity after application. I personally have found lemon essential oil to be mildly irritating to the skin, so test it before applying.

Mint: Use mint as you would lemon: to refresh and awaken the mind, and brighten the mood. Mint leaves are a wonderful addition to magical or moon-blessed water when your intention is to refresh, invigorate, and cleanse, and mint is easy to grow—so easy, in fact, that some gardeners will run away screaming if you offer them mint plants, because they will take over entire areas just like bamboo. If you don't want your entire yard to be a sea of mint, grow it in pots. Mint's vigorous, hardy, rapid growth is a property that lends itself to magical intention for revival and renewal, and a return to health.

Oregano: Another darling of Italian cooks, oregano is rich in antioxidants, and is anti-bacterial, anti-inflammatory, and antiviral. When consumed or applied to the skin, it may even slow the growth of cancer cells.[60] It is effective with inflammatory issues, and is a natural pain reliever. Like basil, it's easy to grow at home, available as an essential oil, and considered safe for the skin when in a carrier oil; however, it is another essential oil that can cause a burning sensation on the skin, so it must

---

60. Rachel Link, "6 Science-Based Health Benefits of Oregano," Healthline.com, last updated October 27, 2017, https://www.healthline.com/nutrition/6-oregano-benefits.

be diluted. Use it fresh or dried, and add it to a sachet or potpourri when a spicy, stimulating, invigorating scent is desired.

Rose: There's nothing quite as iconic for representing true love as a red rose. Like jasmine and lavender, the lovely scent of rose has an immediately soothing effect. Rose can soften and sweeten a relationship, and perk it up if need be. If your Sacred Massage intention is to enrich a romantic relationship, invoke the lovely powers of rose by sprinkling fresh petals, using dried flowers or petals in potpourri, or adding rose essential oil to your massage oil or lotion. Although rose's classic correlation is romantic love, it can also represent deep, binding love for anyone. Love can take many forms. When your magical intention includes deep, true love and a loyal heart, rose has this covered too.

Rosemary: Rosemary is another powerhouse herb, and a hardy and beautiful plant that's easy to grow. The fresh herb is a cook's best friend, and growing your own plant means you'll always have fresh rosemary for those savory dishes. Like oregano and clove, rosemary is stimulating, and is magically associated with protection, health, vigor, purification, and healing. Rosemary is an antioxidant, and supports the immune system, improves memory and concentration when used in aromatherapy, and may provide protection from cancer.[61]

Sage: Burning sage is iconic in the magical community, often used in a wand or cleansing a space, magical tools or surfaces, or even people before entering a magical circle or ritual. For massage, sage smoke could be used to magically cleanse your loved one of negative energy and influences before you begin, or to clear the energy in your massage space before a session. Using sage smoke in this way was once called "smudging," but this is a sacred practice in the indigenous American community, and it's an inappropriate word to use for other purposes, particularly if you aren't a member of that community. A more respectful term is "smoke cleansing." In the non-magical world, sage is considered to be anti-inflammatory and anti-congestive, and particularly helpful for bronchial issues like asthma, bronchitis, and chronic cough.[62] Although a beloved herb in the magical community, the use of white sage is frowned upon by many because it is sacred to the Indigenous American commu-

---

61. WebMD Editorial Contributors, "Health Benefits of Rosemary," WebMD.com, last updated September 18, 2020, https://www.webmd.com/diet/health-benefits-rosemary.

62. WebMD Editorial Contributors, "Are There Health Benefits to Using Sage Oil?" WebMD.com, last updated October 22, 2020, https://www.webmd.com/diet/health-benefits-sage-oil.

nity. Commercial harvesting of wild sage deprives the indigenous community of a sacred herb that they need. If you really want to work with sage, either grow and dry it yourself, or purchase it from an authentic indigenous seller.

Salt: Our favorite table ingredient is magically associated with protection and purification, and used to repel negative energy or define boundaries. You'll remember that a line of salt was suggested after expelling negative energy from your massage area and home to create a magical boundary. There are times when boundaries might be appropriate in massage, like for a loved one who needs protection from something or someone. Salt can also serve as a magical detox if you find yourself saturated in someone else's energy after working on them. Cleanse your energy field by soaking in salted bath water, or rubbing salt over your body in the shower. Much as we care about our loved ones, sometimes we need to scrub their energy off after spending a lot of time with them. It doesn't mean we don't love them. It just means we need a return to emotional equilibrium, where our own energy is ours, and their energy is theirs. A salt bath or shower is a magical "reboot." Epsom salt also does this, but it isn't actually salt. It is a combination of magnesium and sulfate, that easily dissolves in warm water to relax muscles and ease joint pain. It is not meant to be ingested.

Vanilla: Like rose and jasmine, the scent of vanilla is sweet and yummy, often reminding people of the scent of home-baked cookies. If baking cookies don't trigger an immediate rush of pleasure, I don't know what will! When you just want to give your loved one some pure, peaceful pleasure, vanilla is perfect. You can use kitchen vanilla or vanilla beans for magical work, but for massage, use vanilla essential oil in a mist or diffuser, dotted on your table or sheets, or added to massage oil. Side note: There's no such thing as actual pure vanilla essential oil. The "essential oil" is a carrier oil that contains vanilla resin or extract.

Incense

I mention incense mainly as a "fashion don't" for a massage session because, like smoke from candles, incense smoke can irritate lungs, noses, and throats. Also, some people find it too intense or just don't like it. However, incense does have a place for cleansing and dedicating magical spaces, tools, and items, and is a staple in magical work and ritual. If you love incense, use it for magical work outside your massage space, or when no one else will be in the room but you. Incense is great for altars—not so great for massage sessions.

Magical/Moon-Blessed Water

We've established that smoke and massage don't mix, and some people just prefer to cleanse or dedicate something or someone without using smoke. You can do this with magical water or moon-blessed water, which is simple to make yourself. Things you make yourself are magically saturated with your intention and compassion, and you know exactly what's in them, so they are perfect for massage uses. Magical or moon-blessed water is made from water and any herb, leaf, or flower (preferably fresh). Salt may also be used if it aligns with an intention of creating boundaries or purifying. Combine the ingredients in a clear jar or bottle, breathe or speak your intention into the water, and leave the jar out under the light of a full moon for a whole night.

The full moon is iconic in the Pagan world, and a preferred time for powerful magic, spellwork, and ritual that's intended to bring something to full fruition. For massage, decide what you want to bring to full fruition—compassion or healing or relief—and infuse your intention into the water. If you want a little extra full-moon energy, you can do this process as a ritual, right under the light of a full moon.

Altars

An altar isn't just a pretty collection of stuff that makes you happy (even though it usually does just that)—it's an arrangement of thoughtfully, specifically chosen items and symbols intended to attract a specific energy, reinforce your magical intention, or strengthen a divine relationship. It has a job to do! Altars exist in most every spiritual or religious practice, and appear in homes, businesses, outdoors, and in places of worship.

Altars are used for a variety of magical purposes, such as attraction (bringing certain energies toward you), magical work (doing spellwork or serving as a working centerpiece during a ritual), or honoring deity (expressing your appreciation and devotion to a particular deity, which we discussed in the chapter on deity). Altars are also focal points for celebrating a season, event, holiday, or life passage, such as a wedding, new baby, or the arrival of spring. They are also created for remembrance, to honor deceased loved ones and ancestors.

We already explored how your massage table (or the surface you're working on) can serve as your working magical massage altar, and you could leave it at that. However, adding other altars to the room can provide a magical energy boost, and serve as validating, comforting reminders of your own divine magical energy and intention. In addition, you may want to do actual non-massage magical work outside your massage session to support your loved one's health and happiness. For example, you may wish to do a ritual supporting your loved one's recovery from an injury or illness, and leave that altar standing to do its work for as long as you want. However, when creating an altar or performing a ritual for someone else, it's important to have that person's permission before proceeding. In my opinion, doing magic or ritual aimed at creating any change—positive or negative—in another person's life is unethical. You should never assume that you know better than another person what is best for them, no matter how right or logical or beneficial it seems to you.

Altars can be very small and simple, or large and elaborate. You can create them in your massage space or anywhere in your home where you want a focal point for connecting to magical energy, doing magical work or ritual, inspiration, prayer, meditation, contemplation, celebration, remembrance, or worship.

Components of a Magical Altar

Although there are specific magical tools and items typically present on an altar, the most effective altars are those that are meaningful and symbolic to you. Always be genuine, and create from your own heart. Spirit will know if you're faking it, or if you don't really believe in what you're doing. "Copycat magic" is not optimal—or effective—in my opinion, and that goes for altars too. Make all your magical practices your own. That said, for the sake of learning, we'll create a typical magical altar with all the typical features, and if you love them, great! If not—switch it up your own way, and make your own kind of magic. Although your massage table serves as your actual working altar where the healing magic happens, you may wish to create an additional magical altar in your massage room or elsewhere to focus your magical intention or amp up your magical connection to Spirit.

A very basic magical working altar usually includes a candle (or several), incense, and representation of the God and Goddess (or male and female energy), which could be an athame and chalice, or plain old kitchen knife and a wine glass or goblet. There is representation of each of the four elements, as well as Spirit. If a certain deity is desired for that altar's magical purpose, it would be represented by an image, figurine, or symbol of that deity. Crystals, stones, shells, herbs, symbols, and fresh greenery or flowers are also often included on an altar.

Activity
CREATE AN ALTAR

Let's create a simple attraction altar, meant to draw healing energy into your massage work. Before we start, you first need to decide where it belongs. Walk through your house and find a place that calls to you; a spot that feels "just right" for that altar. Cleanse and dedicate this little space just as you did your massage space.

For an altar cloth, choose a cloth in the color that represents your massage intention. Spread the cloth over the altar, and spritz it with some moon-blessed water or an essential oil mist that supports your intention, or magically cleanse it with incense or herbal smoke. From the list of magical crystals, choose one, or some, that best represent the healing, compassionate energy you want. If you don't have that specific crystal, go for a walk and pick up a rock that seems to call to you, or use one you already have, and breathe, scratch, write, or paint your intention onto that rock.

Place a representation of the four elements onto the cloth, preferably at their actual directions. For the grounding, healing, comforting energy of earth, use dirt, rocks, plants, nuts, or seeds, images or figurines forest animals or animals that work the land, and items that are brown or green. For the clearing, refreshing, uplifting energy of air, use feathers, images or figurines of birds, or anything that creates sound, like a bell or chime, and items that are yellow or pastel. For the vigor, vitality, and strength of fire, use a candle, incense, or images or figurines of animals symbolic of fire energy, like scorpions or red stallions, or items that are red or orange. For the calming, loving, flowing energy of water, use seashells or sea glass, images or figurines of fish, mermaids, or the ocean, and items that are blue or purple.

Scratch or breathe your healing intention into a candle, and place that on your altar. From the list of magical herbs and oils, choose one that aligns with your healing intention. You can place dried or fresh herbs there on a little dish, or dot some essential oil here and there. If you'd like to include your healing deity on your altar, place a figurine, image, or symbol associated with that deity there.

You can stop here, or keep on going: adorn your altar with flowers, sparkly beads or glitter scattered here and there, or a string of fairy lights entwined around the items on the altar, or strung above it. You are limited only by your own creativity. Have fun with this activity, and really pour your heart into it. There's no "right" way to do this. Just create a magical assemblage that expresses your unique, genuine self and your magical massage intention.

When you're satisfied with your work, bestow a blessing on your altar, such as, "May healing, love, and compassion flow through my massage sessions," or another phrase or mantra that is meaningful to you and represents your massage intention. Welcome each of the elements to your altar, and also your deity if it is represented there. When you feel satisfied and solid with what you've created, cleanse and dedicate your finished altar like you did your massage table: Spritz it with moon-blessed water, or swirl incense, bay leaf, or sage smoke over it, and chant a dedication mantra, such as "Magic flows through this space." Place your hands on the altar, draw in the divine magical energy of the universe, channel it through your hands, and trace a meaningful symbol on it or over it. Welcome this altar into your massage learning and practice. Finish just as you did when completing the cleansing and dedication of your massage table: place your palms on the altar and say, "So mote it be" or "Amen," or any other word, mantra, or phrase that "seals the deal" and makes it so.

One more note about altars: Their energy is dulled by dirt and dust, so clean them regularly. Also, feel free to change or rearrange your altar if you wish. I usually change my altars around when I clean them. It refreshes their energy. Whenever you clean and/or change your altar, re-cleanse it with smoke, and restate your magical massage intention. You may add things, or take things away, but your love, compassion, and desire to heal will always be a constant.

So Much More About Magic

If you're intrigued by these magical items and practices, there's an entire world of magic to discover. There are multiple books written on just about any magical topic you could imagine. Unless you want to commit to a particular Pagan path and study magic in that tradition, just start exploring, and collect what works for you. Adapt things to a massage focus. And, once again, remember: The stuff doesn't make magic. You do. The stuff just provides a little magical boost to keep you focused on your massage intentions and keep that magical energy flowing.

Chapter 6

Touch Is Magical

In the last chapter, we talked about magical "stuff," and your external experience. Now, we'll turn to magical energy and your internal experience. Without magical energy, will, and determination, magical stuff is just a bunch of cool, sparkly knick-knacks. You can do magic without stuff, but you can't do it without your own focused energy, intention, and implementation. It's like a car. It doesn't matter how cool the car is, it won't go without gas. Your energy and will is your magical gas.

Magic is neither good nor bad. In a way, it's essentially inert, like electricity. Electricity can light your home, but it can also electrocute. It isn't the electricity itself that's helpful or harmful, it's the knowledge and skill of the one using the electricity that makes it one or the other. When you employ magic, you are the power cord. You plug into the electricity, and at the other end of that power cord is your magical goal, or "intention," as well as the specific things you do to set that intention in motion, called "implementation." The final result of that focus and work is the result, or "manifestation." You are the physical element through which this magical energy passes on its way to fulfillment.

Where Magic and Massage Meet

Just after starting massage school, I randomly—and thankfully—toddled onto the Pagan path. Finally, I'd found my tribe, and could exhale and just be my true, genuine self. I was utterly enamored with this magical, mystical community filled with exploration and learning. It was literally a brand-new world, full of wonders and discoveries, and amongst them, my first ritual. It was a joyful public ritual at a festival, focused upon connection and raising magical energy. The very first thing we did was grounding and centering. Well, what a coincidence! Grounding and centering is also the first step in a massage! This opened my mind to the many similarities between magic and massage. Over time, I realized that a massage session is essentially a ritual. This inspired me to continue shaping my massage work into a magical practice.

Magic is part of every massage I do. My client may or may not realize it, because it's very subtle. I'm not chanting or waving wands or swirling smoke over them. It all transpires internally, within my own magical focus. My clients don't notice anything out of the ordinary, other than that I pause and breathe at the beginning and ending of each massage, but they are aware that for that hour, they feel completely and totally nurtured. And they truly are. They aren't just bodies that pass under my hands. I want each client to feel like they are my *only* client—that they have one hundred percent of my attention, care, and concern. I want them to feel like they're my favorite person in the whole world—and for that hour, they are!

There are some things I do for each client, such as inviting Kuan Yin to participate, as well as certain blessings and mantras. However, my focus (intention) and the massage routine itself (implementation) is customized to each person, depending on their needs. One may simply need to relax, while another needs their sore, tight shoulders to be softened and relieved. Sacred Massage is not a "one size fits all" process. It's shaped for each person with thoughtfully, mindfully selected magical practices.

Intention, Implementation, and Manifestation

Magical work is a process of intention, implementation, and manifestation. Intention is what you desire. Implementation is what you do. Manifestation is what you release. We discussed these concepts in general in the last chapter. Now, we'll apply them to massage.

Intention

Magic is a lot like cooking. You don't just throw random things into a bowl—say, grapes, tuna, oatmeal, and ketchup—mix them up, and hope they produce a cake. Yuck! No, first, you decide what you want to make (intention), pick a recipe, and gather the necessary ingredients. Same with massage. With your loved one's needs in mind, you create a specific massage intention (recipe) for your Sacred Massage session: *I will help Melissa relax and breathe. I will soften Steven's tight shoulders. I will provide emotional comfort for Mom.* If your loved one just wants soothing, simple, relaxation, your intention might be more generic: *Relax, rest, and breathe.*

You can also design your intention around whatever healing deity you wish to include in that session: *May Kuan Yin's compassion be present in my touch. I welcome the healing knowledge of Asclepius. I will be a vessel for Yemaya's protective love in this session.* You might also craft your intention to align with an elemental energy, an archangel, the cool, green, growing earth, or the energies of the cosmos and heavenly bodies: *I align myself with the divine healing light of Raphael. Let the flowing love and peace of water carry me through this session.* You could set an intention on an overall focus: *I will channel serenity. Love shall be the source of all that I do. Healing magic will emanate from my hands.* Your intention could even be a simple mantra: *Only healing … Only peace …* Your intention can be just about anything you wish as long as it provides clarity, focus, and meaning to what you're about to do.

If you happen to become distracted while doing your massage, and discover your head is full of unwanted thoughts, you can repurpose your intention like a magical re-set button to clear your mind and focus on what you're doing. I have a particular phrase I think when my mind drifts beyond the walls of my massage office: *Be here now.* That's my well-worn cue to snap back to center, focus, clear, and pay attention to what I'm doing right here, right now, *only.*

Implementation

Intention defines your magical goal, but just picking a recipe and arranging the ingredients on the counter won't bake that cake. You have to actually *do* something. You must combine those ingredients just the right way, put them in the right pan, and set the oven at the right temperature to make that cake happen. This is "implementation"—the specific method you've chosen to make your intention happen.

In massage, implementation begins with the physical massage techniques, which we'll learn later on in detail. Implementation happens when you place your hands on your loved one. Implementation is the *doing.*

Manifestation

Continuing with our baking analogy, you've set your intention and chosen your recipe. You've gathered up all the tools and ingredients, and implemented your intention while mixing everything up, putting it in the pan, and placing it in the oven. But that cake hasn't materialized just yet. Right now, it's just a pan full of sweet slop. The oven will "manifest" your intention. When you pull that pan back out—Yay! Cake! When you release your magical intention to the universe (Spirit), it "bakes your cake." It picks up where you left off, and makes that intention materialize: manifestation.

In massage, manifestation happens as you finish your massage. Your massage techniques and sequences are finished. You're seated, with your loved one's head cradled in your palms. This is the moment for channeling divine love and compassion, bestowing blessings, activating mantras, and clearing away any residual unwanted energy. Your loved one is infused with divine and magical energy. You complete your Sacred Massage session by releasing your intention to Spirit to make it so.

Grounding and Centering

Grounding and centering is usually done before beginning a magical ritual. It clears your mind, reinforces your connection to your body and the earth. If it's a group ritual, everyone might be directed to place their palms on the earth, or breathe slowly and deeply together, or chant the "Om" as one. The group might be led on a guided grounding meditation, such as imagining a cord stretching from your spine down into the core of the earth, connecting to her low, slow, steady, calming vibration. There are myriad ways to approaching grounding and centering, and people choose whichever method works best for them.

"Grounding and centering" are typically phrased together, because they're interconnected, like a two-step process. You ground to connect to the earth and your body, often through your breath, which slows your heartbeat and promotes relaxation. As you relax physically, so do you mentally—your mind is able to loosen its grip on intrusive or stressful thoughts, and just "center" on the experience of being at one with the earth and your body.

In massage, grounding and centering is essentially the same as in a magical ritual: You feel your connection to the earth and your body, and clear your mind to focus on simply being present. No thoughts, no feelings—just *be*-ing. You become comfortably situated in your own body and mind, ready to serve as a clear, open channel for magical energy.

Whether doing magic or massage, grounding aligns your own energetic vibration with the earth's: slow and methodical; cool, calm, and peaceful. Centering means bringing your mind into relaxed, clear focus, and dispelling any unwanted thoughts that may be swirling around in your head. You ground and then center as one smooth process. When you're calm and clear, you're ready to begin doing magical work (implementation), whether in ritual or your massage space.

Activity
GROUNDING AND CENTERING MEDITATION

This meditation cues you to simply ground and center. Rather than attempt to simultaneously read and do this meditation (which is literally impossible because your mind can't be clear and focused if words are streaming through it, or out of your mouth), record the meditation on your phone and play it back to yourself, or have someone read it to you while you do the meditation. Don't just gallop through it. Pause at the end of each sentence, allowing yourself time to align with the words.

Choose a time and place when you won't be disturbed. Get comfortable, get all the wigglies out, and then focus on your breathing, into and out of your belly button. With each breath, go a little slower and deeper, but don't force it—only relaxed, comfortable, effortless breath, like ocean waves rolling in and out.

As you breathe, relax and clear your mind. Acknowledge any intrusive thoughts, and send them away in a pink bubble.

Turn your attention to the part of your body making contact with the earth and her gravity. If you're sitting in a chair, that might be your feet; if lying down, the length of your whole body. Really *feel* Mother Earth's gravitational pull. Lift an arm, and then let it flop down limp. It's not just falling—that is Earth's gravity pulling it back. You are quite literally grounded to her.

Sink into the experience of Mother Earth pulling you close. Take comfort in that protective power. She is holding you tight. Nothing can harm you here. You are completely safe. Tell yourself, "I am safe." Relax into Mother Earth's calm, comforting safety.

When you feel comfortably grounded and connected to Mother Earth, turn your attention to your breath, flowing freely and effortlessly. Experience the calm emptiness of your mind.

Think or say, "I am safe…I am peaceful…I am present." Let the words just tumble though your mind or from your lips, as many times as you wish.

Return your focus to your breath, and relax in this grounded, centered experience for as long as you wish.

Open your eyes, and return to where you began.

Walk around with It, Put It On

Do this meditation again, but this time at the end, instead of returning to where you began, hold onto that grounded, centered feeling as you open your eyes, and maintain this simultaneously calm and alert state, completely present in that precise moment in time and nowhere else. Stand up and walk around, still alertly grounded and centered in that present moment. If you have an energetic wobble or distraction, recall the phrases from the meditation: *I am safe … I am peaceful … I am present.* Visualize this feeling of calm alertness as a cozy sweater, and in your mind, put it on. Feel its warmth, softness, and comfort.

Linking feelings with images is one of the components of neuro-linguistic programming, or NLP,[63] and this sort of detailed visualization and precise imagery are also components of magic. In time, this NLP process allows you to easily recall that alert calmness by just imagining the sweater and putting it on. You can wear it right into your massage session or put it on whenever you wish. NLP is also useful for magically charging and dedicating a magical tool.

Activity
IMAGINE GROUNDING AND CENTERING

In a massage session, grounding and centering begins when you place your hands on your loved one's body—their earth—for the first time. There is no movement. Only touch.

Imagine that you're standing beside your loved one, lying facedown on a massage table, covered with a sheet. You're facing them, about to place your palms on their back. You don't just plop your hands onto someone's body like you're about to knead dough. No. You intentionally, mindfully *place* your palms on their back. Your very first touch—over the sheet or clothing, before beginning any massage techniques—is a kinesthetic communication: *Everything is fine. You are completely safe. You can relax.* With that touch, you are grounding to your loved one's "earth"—their body. Be open to whatever energy is happening there. No judgment, just awareness.

Imagine your palms resting on your loved one's back, relax, breathe deeply and effortlessly, and feel the solid ground beneath your feet. Breathe in, and exhale

---

63. GoodTherapy, "Neuro-Linguistic Programming (NLP)," GoodTherapy.org, accessed March 18, 2022, https://www.goodtherapy.org/learn-about-therapy/types/neuro-linguistic-programming.

any unnecessary or distracting thoughts, feelings, or energy down through your legs, through the soles of your feet, right into the earth. Feel your connection to the earth and inhale that slow, steady vibration of the earth. Imagine it rising up through your feet and legs, up through your body and arms, and on through your palms to your loved one.

Inhale deeply, and breathe that grounding earth energy right through your palms, and into your loved one. Relax your hands to the curvature of their body, noticing the warmth coming through the sheet. Send some warming energy back through your soft, relaxed hands. There's no pressure, only comforting contact. As you breathe, continue channeling earth's calming, low vibration back and forth through your palms, as if you're inhaling and exhaling right through your loved one and the earth, like a living two-way channel of calm, grounded energy.

Center your mind by swiping away any unnecessary thoughts, and focusing upon that present moment only. There's no past, no future. Only the present moment. Recall that feeling of calm alertness from the meditation and let it fill you up. Think a "present moment only" mantra for grounding and centering. Mine is: "Be here now. You have nowhere to be but here." That mantra is an instant prompt to release everything outside the room and inside my mind, and just be present in that moment.

Grounded and centered, calm and alert, recall your magical intention, and proceed with implementation.

Magical Massage Implementation

After grounding and centering, implementation begins with inviting the four cardinal directions, and the elemental energies associated with them. A deity, or several, are often invited next, as well as the God and Goddess. Some in the magical community prefer the word "invoke," but I find this word quite impudent and presumptuous when addressing divine or elemental energy. I prefer to "invite" or "welcome."

Inviting the Elements, and God and Goddess

We touched upon the four directions and some of their energies for your massage table dedication ritual and in the activity for creating a magical altar. Let's take it a few steps further.

Imagine the directions as four points on a circle, spaced equally, like points on a cross. Each direction is associated with an element, and its symbolism and energies:

North: Earth, the body, physical health, wealth, caves, soil, rocks, the fields and forests, forest animals.

East: Air, the mind, thoughts, intelligence, learning, strategy, the high mountain peaks and sky, wind, flying animals.

South: Fire, the will, courage, power, stamina, sexuality, charisma, the hot, dry deserts, and lava and volcanos, animals that sting, bite, or strike.

West: Water, the emotions, creativity, love, compassion, serenity, all bodies of water, animals that live in water.

The fifth element, positioned in the center of these four quarters, is Spirit: divinity, intuition, purity, connection, one's own true self. Sometimes this element is invoked in ritual, sometimes not. Sometimes the God and Goddess—representing the balance of divine male/projective and divine female/receptive energies—are invoked at this point. As in most things Pagan, different people and different groups do things different ways. In Sacred Massage, we'll freestyle a bit.

One of the super cool things about massage is that all the elements are already present in the process: earth is the body; air is breath; fire heats your palms; water flows through the movement of your hands over the body; Spirit channels through you to your loved one. The God and Goddess are also inherently represented in the massage process: you project healing energy, and your loved one receives it.

In a magical ritual, the leader (or an appointee) would walk to each direction or face it, and formally welcome the element associated with that direction. In massage, this process can be done mentally, just after grounding and centering. To welcome the elements mentally, turn your mind or tip your head toward each cardinal direction and its associated elements, welcoming them one at a time, beginning at north and moving clockwise. Welcome Spirit after the four directional elements, returning your focus to center. Mentally welcome the God and Goddess. For massage, we keep the ritual steps quick, clean, and simple, rather than the usual ceremonial pomp and circumstance. We want things to flow quietly—physically, spiritually, and magically. Although you are beginning your magical massage ritual internally, your loved one is only aware that you are both taking a moment to breathe and settle into this peaceful, quiet moment together.

Activity
IMAGINE INVITING DIVINE ENERGY AND DEITY

Recalling your earlier activity, where you imagined grounding and centering, imagine you are still standing with your palms on your loved one's back. After inviting the elements, and God and Goddess, you next invite the healing deity you've chosen for your Sacred Massage sessions. Call to them in your mind. Open up to their energy and welcome it inside you, and into your session. Let your gratitude for this participation flow toward that deity. In your mind, repeat the mantra or phrase you chose or created to align with that deity: *May the healing magic of Isis be ever present.* If you don't want to work with deity, you could substitute meaningful energy, such as healing pink light, and create a meaningful phrase to represent that energy: *May I be filled with the pink light of love.*

As the mantra or phrase passes through your mind, you simultaneously slide your palms slowly apart down the spine, very gently, one hand resting at the base of the neck, the other on the slope of the hips. Imagine that you're spreading that phrase or mantra right over your loved one's back, infusing them with that message. You can also use this message to serve as a refocusing prompt should you become distracted by anything that "isn't here now."

Ritual

Grounding and centering, and inviting divine energy and deity, begin the implementation process in a magical ritual. In part three, we'll learn the physical tools, techniques, and sequences of Soothing Touch, which implement your magical massage intention. Manifestation happens when we bring everything together for a complete Sacred Massage session. A Sacred Massage session is organized like a magical ritual and, in fact, is a ritual. We'll learn a basic template for magical ritual next, and revisit it when we learn the Sacred Massage sequence/ritual.

Ritual simply means "doing a particular thing a particular way for a particular reason at a particular time." It might be magical, it might not be. If you've ever been to a wedding, graduation, or funeral, you've been to a ritual, and may have already participated in one. A magical ritual can be just about anything you could imagine, from an initiation to spellwork to celebrating an accomplishment to heralding a change of seasons. It can be wildly elaborate or something as simple as meditating on a phrase or image. A massage session can also be structured and performed as a ritual.

In addition to doing massage as a ritual, there are other ways you might find ritual useful, such as formally dedicating a space or item and infusing it with magical energy. You might also do a ritual for yourself, maybe to acknowledge yourself as a healer, or when facing a difficult massage issue, such as a loved one undergoing cancer treatment or facing end-of-life issues—those situations when simple rest and relaxation aren't enough.

Although you could drop everything and do a ritual on the spot in a pinch, without any planning or tools, it's a much more satisfying experience to plan it in advance and really make it a special and meaningful occasion for a celebration, transition, or accomplishment, or for extra healing energy. If you want to include an altar in your ritual, you would also plan this in advance, and have the altar assembled and any necessary items such as matches or a pen and paper already handy. It's a bummer to get yourself magically energized and prepared, go to your altar in the center of your already-cast magical circle, and realize you don't have matches to light the incense and candles.

Certain magical tools are typically used in ritual (and often included on an altar, as we learned), such as a wand or athame (magical ritual knife) to direct energy and represent the God and projective energy, and a chalice or goblet to represent the Goddess and receptive energy. However, your hands can replace these tools in ritual, as they are the conduit for massage magic, healing, and divine, sacred energy. The index finger of your right hand becomes your athame or wand, because the right half of the body is associated with projective energy, and your cupped left hand becomes your chalice, because the left half of the body is associated with receptive energy.

Ritual Begins with Intention

The first step for planning any ritual is to clearly define your intention. You can't get where you want to go if you don't know where you want to go! Make your intention specific. "I want Grandpa to feel better" isn't specific enough. "I will ease Grandpa's low back pain" is better. You don't want to leave the interpretation of your intention up to the universe, because you might not get the answer you were imagining. Grandpa might end up with a case of whiskey on his doorstep, and that might definitely make him feel better, but it won't do a thing for his low back pain.

If you want to do more than just state your intention, you could write a quatrain, which is a four-lined poem in which either the first two sentences and second two sentences rhyme, or the first and third, and the second and fourth. It's often spoken as a magical chant. This quatrain can literally be anything, as long as it captures your intention. It can be flowery and formal, or simple and straightforward: *My Grandpa hurts. His back is tight. Healing hands, make it right.*

Some magical practitioners like to repeat the quatrain three or nine times, speaking ever-increasing energy into the words. Others prefer not to use quatrains, and speak directly and spontaneously from the heart. As in all things magic, do whatever feels genuine and meaningful to you.

Moon Phase

Another basic ritual consideration is the phase of the moon, with which you'll time your ritual. If your intention is to pull healing energy toward you or your loved one, plan your ritual during the waxing or full moon. The full moon is considered to be the most powerfully saturated time to do magic or ritual. If your intention is to push pain, disease, or illness away from you or your loved one, plan it during the waning moon. If it's a dark/new moon, skip over that day. Dark moon magic isn't really a "101" practice, and is generally not particularly congruent with massage. However, it is a good time for turning inward and focusing on what's troubling you.

Ritual Template

This basic ritual template will familiarize you with the steps and flow of a typical magical ritual. This template is simple, like a child's coloring book, as opposed to the oil masterpiece of a magical ritual performed by a master magician. We'll return to this template and repurpose it for Sacred Massage in the "Touch Is Sacred" chapter.

Cleansing/Purifying: Clear stale or negative energy from the space with incense or herbal smoke, or with sound, such as a bell or tuning fork, or your own voice. Because we're focusing on Sacred Massage, you might use your magical hands to cleanse the area by clapping away any negative or unhelpful energy or sweeping it up and away, using your hands for a broom and dustpan, just as you did for your massage area.

Grounding/Centering: Ground yourself to the earth and your body, and clear your mind of unhelpful thoughts. Breathe. Open your crown chakra to receive the divine healing love of the universe and imagine it streaming pure white light through your crown and on down through your body, especially to your arms and hands. Allow a circle of warmth and energy to build in the center of your palms.

Circle Casting: A magical circle is cast to create a protective energetic dome. Helpful, supportive energies may enter the dome, and harmful, negative energies may not. Stand at north, point your index finger at the ground, and imagine Spirit's pure white light streaming from your fingertip to the ground. Walk a clockwise circle all the way back to north. Your circle is cast.

Calling Energies and Deities: Move or turn to the north, and welcome its energies: *"Welcome, North—earth, healing, rest, cool green forests, and protective caves."* Walk or turn clockwise, pausing at each cardinal direction, and do the same. Invite the deities you want to participate, and welcome them. Treat the energies and deities with respect, not as servants you're commanding to be present. (Some people prefer to invite archangels in place of the directions or elements.)

Invite and welcome the energies of the God and Goddess by holding up your projective right index finger (God) and receptive cupped left hand (Goddess), and symbolize the union of these energies by placing your right finger in your left palm. Treats are usually offered to the God and Goddess in ritual to express gratitude for their participation. The classic "cakes and ale" are typically cake or cookies and wine, or something a particular deity really loves, like honey or fruit. These offerings are not meant to be consumed. They are left on the altar, and when spent or when the altar is dismantled, emptied under a favorite bush or tree.

Raise Energy: Spark up magical energy inside your magical dome by dancing, singing, chanting, clapping, or drumming. Let yourself go and really get those magical juices flowing. When you feel energized, you're ready to get to work.

Magical Work: This is the heart of the ritual, and of implementation. Stand at your altar, and light the candle or incense. State your intention or recite your quatrain. Say or do anything else that is meaningful to you, such as singing a song, playing a musical instrument, or doing a meditation. Restate your intention, adding, "For the greater good of all and with harm to none."

Conclude your statement with a confident "So mote it be!" With that, you direct all the energy you raised and your implementation out to the universe, like a beam of light. And then, let it go. Manifestation is not up to you—it's up to the universe. Summon a feeling of complete confidence, absolutely *knowing* that your intention *will* be manifested. "So mote it be" is a traditional phrase said to end a magical working or ritual, and essentially means, "May it be so" or "I will it to be so." It's the Pagan equivalent to "Amen." And if you'd rather say, "Amen," that's okay too.

Thank the Energies and Deities: Express heartfelt gratitude to any deities that participated in your ritual, as well as the God and Goddess, and wish them "Hail and farewell." Face north and thank the energies, wishing them "Hail and farewell." Moving or turning counterclockwise this time, walk to each cardinal direction and do the same.

Uncasting the Circle: Beginning at north, point your index finger to the circle of white light you cast, and vacuum that light back into your finger as you walk the circle counterclockwise, vacuuming all the way, and returning to north. The veil between the magical and mundane worlds has dissolved, and all is as it was when you began.

Farewell: In a public ritual, a song might be sung or gratitude to participants expressed. Often there's a traditional joyful collective shout of "Merry meet, merry part, and merry meet again." This just means we meet joyfully, part joyfully, and will be joyful when we gather again. When working on your own, you can do whatever feels appropriate at this point: a song, a poem, some quiet meditation.

Celebration: After a ritual comes refreshments. People like to hang out afterwards and socialize, and enjoy refreshments. If you're doing a solo ritual (called "solitary"), celebrate your magical accomplishment with a cup of tea, glass of wine, or whatever makes you feel special—after all, you just communed with divine energy!

Magic and Energy

Magic requires an awareness of the divine energy of the universe or Spirit, and inviting it to flow through your ritual or magical work. The universe responds by manifesting your intention. That response may be very subtle. You have to listen carefully for it. For example, if you did a ritual to find a new apartment, the response may be a gut feeling to drive a different route to work, or even being rerouted due to street construction, and passing by a complex with a "Now Renting" banner hanging across the front. The universe rarely responds in a huge, flamboyant way, and won't likely drop a new apartment in front of you from out of the sky. The response comes in clues, intuitions, or serendipities that point toward fulfillment of your magical intention.

Magic tells the universe, "I want to get to Chicago," and it responds with road signs: *Turn here. Turn there.* The universe guides you in that direction, rather than serving as the Great Samantha Stevens in the Sky, wiggling your nose and blinking you there. It doesn't do the work for you. You still have to put in the effort, and pay attention to the road signs, clues, intuitions, and serendipities that pop up. A magical mind notices these signs, rather than ignoring them like background noise or writing them off as irrelevant or nonsense. Those who refuse to believe in magic have had unimpressive experiences with it because they've stubbornly stuck to their own definition of what magical manifestation is. As if wearing blinders, they ignored the road signs pointing them toward the manifestation highway.

Magical Massage Energy

Energy is the core of magical work and massage too, particularly energy-intensive modalities like Reiki and Healing Massage. It's the heart of Sacred Massage as well. Your focused intention to channel love, compassion, healing, and relaxation is really all about directing energy—magic, in other words.

I love Christopher Penczak's comments on magic and healing in his book *Magic of Reiki*: "Ultimately, magic is partnering with the universe to create change."[64] Well, isn't that essentially what we're doing in Sacred Massage? Partnering with the divine healing energy of the universe to create physical and emotional change in another person? Pretty spot-on, if you ask me.

In massage, your hands are the conduit for the magical energy of your intention. You draw in divine healing energy from the universe and, of course, mentally direct it toward your loved one. But you also transmit that energy physically through your touch, and create that change Penczak spoke of. Your hands are the divine transmitters of magical, healing energy.

The Hamsa

A magical symbol that symbolizes the divine nature of your hands is the hamsa. It actually *is* a hand—an open palm, sometimes with elaborate decorations or symbols. This ancient Middle Eastern amulet traces back to the area of Tunisia and the northern coast of Africa once known as Carthage. The symbol is traditionally worn or displayed by those of the

---

64. Christopher Penczak, *Magic of Reiki: Focused Energy for Healing, Ritual, and Spiritual Development* (Woodbury, MN: Llewellyn Publications, 2007), 6.

Jewish and Muslim faiths but has broadened out across cultures in recent years. It is also called the Hand of God, Hand of Miriam (Jewish), and the Hand of Fatima (Muslim).

Regardless of culture or religion, the hamsa is a protective talisman, and sometimes has the "nazar" symbol of protection from the evil eye on the palm. If it is a Hand of Miriam, it may have the Star of David in the center. The hamsa attracts health, happiness, and good fortune. When the fingers point up, it is focused upon protection. When pointing down, it is focused upon good fortune, abundance, and positive outcomes.

Hamsas can be found on all sorts of things, from jewelry to home decor. They make perfect visual reminders of the magic you possess in your heart and hands. With health and happiness amongst its central attributes, the hamsa is a meaningful and appropriate spiritual symbol for reinforcing the divine blessings that emanate from your very own hands.

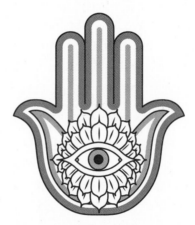

FIGURE 2: HAMSA AND NAZAR

Activity
FEEL THE ENERGY IN YOUR HANDS

You don't need formal Reiki training to detect energy with your hands and move it, or to see energy fields, or auras. Detecting energy takes a little practice because, like magic, these sensations and visions are subtle. One of the first lessons, whether Reiki or magic, is to feel energy between your hands. Give it a try:

Rub your palms together briskly until they're hot, then hold them about a body width apart. Slowly bring your palms together until you feel a thickening in the air. For me, this feels about the size and shape of a grapefruit.

Lightly bounce your hands all around that thick ball of energy so you really detect the change in the air pressure. Play with it. Imagine that you can push this ball away from you and then pull it back. When you're all done playing with it, clap your hands and return this energy to the universe like a sparkly spray of light.

After playing with an energy ball, you may notice that your palms are very warm. You'll notice the same thing when doing massage on your loved one. Sure, your hands become warm because you're using them, but you'll notice that the warmth is particularly concentrated in the center of the palm. This is the spot where healing energy emanates from you toward your loved one, and is also a chakra, or energy whorl.

If you didn't feel a thing after trying this, don't despair. Feeling energy is very subtle. Learning to detect it is like learning to ride a bike. It takes a lot of practice, and failures, before you "get it." And, if you remember learning to ride a bike, you may remember that if you tried too hard, and over-concentrated and got all stiff, you fell over. Once you learned to relax, you smoothly and easily peddled away.

If you didn't feel the energy ball this time, try again another time. In addition to practice, part of detecting energy between the hands—or anywhere else, for that matter—includes relaxing and calming your mind. You can't detect external energy if your mental energy is ricocheting off the walls of your skull like a trapped hummingbird. You must calm the static energy in your own mind to become sensitive to energy outside your own body or in others.

Activity
MEDITATION FOR ENERGIZING YOUR HANDS

Now that you've played with energy a little, let's really embrace our hands as sources for transmitting healing energy. As with the previous meditation, it's preferable to record this meditation and play it back to yourself or have someone read it to you. You could also remember the sequence by assigning each step with a finger, which we also practiced earlier. To recall each step, move that finger slightly and remember the name of the step, which I've put in parentheses.

As always, find a quiet place and time for your meditation, close the door if necessary, and turn off all phones and devices. Sit or lie down, get as comfortable as possible, get all the wigglies out, and proceed.

Turn your attention to the surface you're sitting or lying on, and feel its comforting support. Notice how safe you feel. Nothing can harm you here (thumb: grounding).

Focus on your breathing. Inhale through your nose, and just let the air flow back out easily. Let your breathing deepen, soften, and slow naturally. Imagine the breath coming into and out of your navel, effortlessly. If any unhelpful or unwanted thoughts intrude, capture them in a bubble and release them to the cosmos (index finger: breathing and centering).

Imagine a beam of pure white light emanating from far out in the universe, and streaming through the top of your head (the crown chakra), and filling your entire body with divine, white light. Inhale that white light and exhale it down your arms and into your palms. As the light concentrates in your palms, imagine a ball of orange light forming there, like the glow of an ember. Pause here and focus upon that warm, orange energy building and swirling in your palms (middle finger: light and warmth).

Bring your palms together, gathering that warm energy into a ball, and pull it toward your sternum. Open your palms and press the warm energy into your heart. Let the warmth flow outward through your entire body and fill it up. Think or say a simple phrase or mantra, such as "Healing warmth, healing hands," or just bask in that soft, warm glow (ring finger: spread the warmth).

Turn your focus back to your hands to finish the meditation. Rub them slowly together and around each other, as if massaging that warmth in. Open your eyes and look at these conduits of divine healing energy; these are hands that heal. Say to yourself out loud, "Healing hands … sacred hands." Place your palms together as if in prayer, and finish with a word, phrase, or mantra of your choice. A simple "Namaste" would do nicely (pinky finger: healing hands, sacred hands).

After your meditation, treat your hands to some lovely, scented lotion or oil, or some nurturing coconut or olive oil. Rub it all in, even into the cuticles and fingernails, taking notice of how the muscles, tendons, and bones of each hand feel. Look at your hands carefully and intently, as if you'd never seen them before. Notice something you never noticed before, maybe a freckle or line on your palm. Think about the infinite number of things your hands can do. They really are miraculous. They really are sacred. View and treat them as such.

Chakras

Chakras are whorls of energy at specific places along the torso, neck, head, and just above the head. There are more than one hundred chakras throughout the body, but the main ones are the six that run along the spine from the tailbone to the head, and the seventh just above the head. Each one is associated with particular energies and symbolism, and even particular illnesses or afflictions, as well as a symbol and name.

Although chakras, and the discussion of them, are ubiquitous in our culture, their origin goes back as far as 1500—500 BC, to the sacred Vedic texts of India, the birthplace of yoga. Opening the chakras and connecting to them is part of yoga, as well as meditation, magic, and massage.

Just as you felt that energy ball between your hands, you can feel a dome of energy over the chakras of your loved one's body. While opening yourself up as a vessel for divine energy, hover your palm over each chakra, gently lowering it like a feather until you feel that sensation of an energy ball. The dome over some chakras will feel firm, round, and robust, while others may feel weak, flat, or flimsy.

Open and flowing chakras can be felt many inches away from the body, while those that are closed or sluggish might only be felt a scant inch away from the body. Clear, flowing chakras means healthy energy can travel easily through the body. Blocked energy at a chakra indicates stagnation in the areas associated with that chakra. You don't "heal" these chakras; you "massage" the energy over them to free them up, like pumping a little air into a flat tire. But remember, you aren't the air—you're only the tube through which it passes. The air itself is divine healing energy.

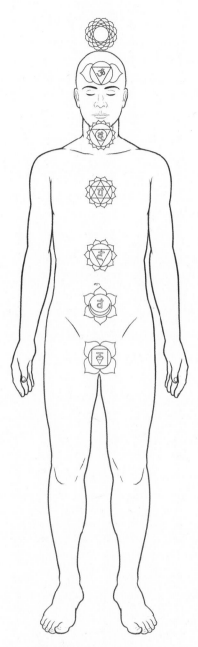

FIGURE 3: CHAKRA FIGURE

These are the seven main chakras, their associations, and their Sanskrit names in parentheses. Certain phrases and mantras are often associated with each chakra, depending on which source or tradition you refer to. The mantras included here are my own.

Root (Muladhara): Located at the base of the spine between the tailbone and pubic bone, the first chakra is the foundation of our feeling of security, safety, and stability. It symbolizes connection to family and tribe. It is the locus of survival, and is depicted in red. Feelings of fear or anxiety are associated with a sluggish root chakra. Its mantra is "I connect."

Sacral (Svadhishthana/Svadisthana/Swadhisthana): Located on the lower abdomen, just above the pubic bone, the second chakra is the source of creative and sexual energy, as well as pleasure. It is the locus of joy, and is depicted in orange. Blocked creativity, or sexual dysfunction or disinterest, are associated with a sluggish sacral chaka. Its mantra is "I enjoy."

Solar Plexus (Manipura): Located at the navel, the third chakra is the powerhouse. It energizes confidence, curiosity, and willpower. It is the locus of momentum, and is depicted in yellow. Weak self-control or willpower and lethargy are associated with a sluggish solar plexus chakra. Its mantra is "I can."

Heart (Anahata): Located at the sternum, near the heart, the fourth chakra is the source of love and empathy, both for others and for oneself, as well as compassion and kindness. It is the locus of love, and is depicted in green. (Some modern traditions associate pink with the Heart Chakra, but the original color is green.) Poor self-esteem, lack of compassion or kindness, hostile or hateful feelings, stressful relationships, suicidal thoughts, depression, or grief can all be associated with a sluggish Heart Chakra. Its mantra is "I love."

Throat (Vishuddha): Located at the center of the throat—right at the larynx, which produces sound for speech—the fifth chakra is the source of clear, effective communication, both spoken and written. It facilitates courage to express our true thoughts or feelings. It is the locus of communication, and is depicted in sky blue, or cyan. Poor communication skills, fear of public speaking or expressing one's true feelings, and chronic dishonesty or deception are associated with a sluggish throat chakra. Its mantra is "I communicate."

Third Eye (Ajna): Located in the center of the forehead, just above and between the eyebrows, the sixth chakra is the locus of intuition, insight, and wisdom, and is depicted in deep purple or indigo. The sixth chakra is the "sixth sense" chakra, allowing one to see what can't be seen. An inability to understand anything beyond the tangible or physical, and poor intuitive skills are associated with a sluggish third eye chakra. Its mantra is "I know."

Crown (Sahasrara): Located just above the top of the head, the seventh chakra is the locus for divine connection, spirituality, and higher consciousness. In meditation, it is often imagined as the portal through which divine energy flows into us. Our own egos can get in the way of this energy, such as when we think we know better than Spirit which path to take or decision to make. Disinterest in or rejection of spirituality or divinity, as well as a disconnection from them, are associated with a sluggish crown chakra. Its color is traditionally lavender; however, it is also depicted as a clear prism, emanating the colors of the rainbow. I prefer the latter because I view this chakra as the prism through which pure, white divine light passes, illuminating the colors of all the other chakras, just like a real prism or crystal hanging in the window—light comes in, and the colors of the rainbow emanate out. Its mantra is "I am," a statement of pure, divine, eternal existence.

Activity
FINDING AND CLEARING THE CHAKRAS

Find an open-minded volunteer, and ask them to lie on their back, relaxed and calm. Both of you can breathe first, and relax. Hover your palm over the root chakra, feel that dome of energy, and define its edge by pulling your palm slowly up and down ever so slightly, an inch or less. Let divine energy flow through you and into that chakra. Don't rush, don't strain. Imagine channeling healing and fresh energy to that chakra. When you feel ready, lift your palm away from the chakra and then slowly and gently lower it to assess whether you detect a change in the dome. It may feel higher and wider. Move up the spine to the next chakra, and repeat this process for each chakra, continuing on up through the crown chakra. If a chakra's energy feels flat or sluggish, it might be a clue about physical or emotional struggles this person is experiencing.

You Are a Magical Conduit

At this point in our massage journey, you're familiar with some spiritual and magical components of Sacred Massage. You may not be proficient with them—yet—but you have the information you need to proceed to the heart of implementation: physical massage techniques. Before we move on, let's recap.

Your hands are a conduit for divine healing and magical energy, but *you* are actually the true conduit. These energies must channel through you before arriving at your hands, to be released toward your loved one. And here's the real kicker: You've always had this ability, you just might not have been aware of it. Now you are. You didn't get a crown chakra after reading this chapter. You've always had one. You aren't a healer because you're reading this book. You're a healer already.

The secret for being a conduit for divine and magical healing energy is that the less you try, the more it moves through you effortlessly. You don't need to force it. It's not a workout. It's not a competition. You only need to be open and welcoming to that divine, magical, healing current, invite it in, and then, just get out of its way. Let it move you, and let it flow. Spirit leads, and you follow. What a gentle, beautiful, magical dance.

PART THREE

The Practice of Soothing Touch

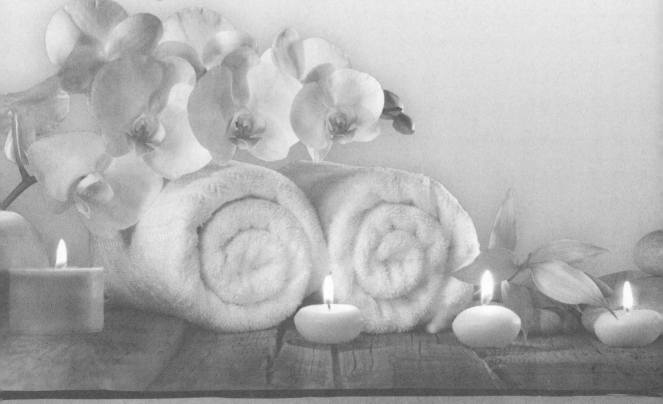

Chapter 7

The Tools and Techniques of Touch

Let's reintroduce you to your own hands. They're so familiar, you probably don't think about them much. They're so available and reliable, you don't have to! You already know myriad ways to use your hands; however, they're capable of even more. Let's expand your relationship with your own hands as we learn the tools and techniques of Soothing Touch.

Swiss Army Hands

"Handy." It means someone or something that can do anything, anytime, anyplace. It's easy to see the root of the word: hand. You know what's really handy? A Swiss Army knife! And your hands are biological Swiss Army knives—they can perform just about any task. Swiss Army hands!

Although there are all sorts of fancy massage tools available, from warm stones to vibrating massage guns, your hands are really the only massage tools you need. Gadgets and gizmos are fun and often very effective, and there's no harm in using them. But your own two loving, amazing, talented hands are all the tools you really need to provide a wonderful, relaxing massage.

Activity
EXPLORING YOUR HANDS ANEW

Take a look at your hands as if you'd never seen them before. Clap them together. Rub the palms briskly together and notice how warm and tingly they get. Spread the fingers open wide and stretch them outward at every point as far as you can.

Ball them into a fist. Squeeze tight. Then relax. Rotate your thumbs around in circles and explore their movement and strength.

With palms facing each other, place the finger pads of one hand on the matching finger pads of the other. Tense your hands and fingers, and release, noticing the strength of the fingers. Press as hard as you can stand, then release the pressure until the fingertips are barely touching, as light as a whisper. There's such a wide spectrum of movement, pressure, and power in your hands and fingers, and such precision. Your hands are miraculous healing "tools," with which you'll make a sacred, soothing connection to a loved one. Through them, you channel the divine, healing energy of your healing deity and the universe, as well as your magical intention.

Slide your thumb along the natural curve of the palm of your opposite hand. Place your thumb on the knuckle at the base of the thumb, and probe all around it. Notice the strong muscles, and how the joint and bones feel. Slide your thumb up to the knuckle at the base of your index finger, and probe that spot, and do the same for each finger, noticing the feel of the bones, joints, and muscles. Probe your palm, and contract and release that hand, feeling the muscles move.

Squeeze the web between your thumb and first finger, probing for a tight band that feels surprisingly tender. When you find it, stop and squeeze hard until the pressure becomes painful. This small but powerful muscle is in constant use, gripping, squeezing, and using scissors or tools. This tender spot is one of many trigger points in the body, and is associated with relieving headaches. A trigger point is a tight, painful spot (we commonly call them "knots"), and can occur in connective tissue (fascia) or in muscles. Trigger points are relieved by deep sustained pressure from thumbs, knuckles, or elbows. Pinch that trigger point again, squeeze hard, and slowly count to thirty. See if this creates some relief and relaxation in your hand, and if you happen to have a headache, count to sixty. See if there's a difference.

The muscles in our hands are constantly working, which can create wear and tear over time on the knuckles. We don't realize it until later in life when arthritis starts to prick those spots. With your thumb and forefinger, squeeze each of the knuckles at the base of your thumb, hold, then squeeze the next knuckle, and finally the tip, right on the nail. Repeat on each finger. Surprise! That feels good, doesn't it?

Play with your hands—push, pull, warm them up, shake them out, let them flap and flop from the wrists. Your hands probably feel super awesome right about now—energized, relaxed, and awake. Whenever your hands feel tired or sore, move them in ways you normally don't, and do a little self-massage on them. Pamper your hands and indulge them with some lotion or oil when you're watching TV. Take care of them. They help you connect with the Divine, and allow you to make massage magic. Treat them like they're precious—because they are!

So Touchy

Let's explore the sensations you can make with your hands and fingers. Even though you may not ultimately use them all in your massage sessions, try them anyway. You might use some, but not others, but should you ever need to do these techniques, they'll be familiar.

You'll practice these moves and techniques on yourself in this chapter before trying on someone else in the following chapters. When practicing on the forearm, rest it on a tabletop, chair arm, or your thigh so it's stable. When practicing on the thigh, sit so the knee is bent and the sole of your foot flat on the ground.

Activity
TECHNIQUES OF TOUCH

Practice the following massage techniques, and with each repetition, play with the speed and the amount of pressure you use. Figure out the range of possibilities for each technique. Get familiar and comfortable with each one before moving on. Find the "too much" point for them. This isn't an exhaustive list of massage techniques—just the "greatest hits" of basic massage moves.

Brushing

Drag your relaxed fingertips lightly along the inside of your forearm, from the wrist to the crook of the elbow, paying attention to the sensations. Repeat on the top of the forearm. Compare the subtle difference in sensation from the same stimulation. Brushing the length of the body over the massage sheet to begin a massage is a nice way to say "hello" to that body, or any area you're about to work on. It's also a gentle way to finish working on an area, or to finish the front or back of the body.

Friction

Friction is briskly rubbing your palm, fist, or "karate chop" side of the hand quickly and briskly back and forth to increase circulation and wake an area up. Try some friction on your forearm with all three hand positions: your palm, then fist, then side of the hand. Go up and down your forearm, and then back and forth across it. It should make your forearm feel tingly and warm.

Gliding and Sliding/Effleurage

Place your palm on top of your thigh, and slide it slowly and smoothly down to the knee, as if spreading dough. Repeat, while leaning onto the heel of your hand, and notice the difference. On your forearm, glide your palm up the underside of your forearm and back down along the top. Let your hand glide smoothly, as if spreading oil. Play with the speed and depth, or "pressure," of gliding and sliding. With this technique, the goal is to go slowly.

Gliding and sliding is called "effleurage" in Swedish massage, and is a basic, gentle technique, commonly used to begin or end a massage session, or a sequence on a certain area of the body. You can glide or slide whenever you want to slow down, or just give a certain area a little more attention. When applying oil or lotion, don't just squirt it onto the body. Squirt it into your palms, and glide and slide it over the skin, warming the area up, using one hand or both.

Grinding

Make a fist, and using the second (middle) row of knuckles, grind them in circles on the top of your thigh. Move the circles around and cover the whole surface of the thigh. Next, place the knuckles into the top of the thigh near the hip, and lean in deeply. Lift, move the knuckles an inch or so toward the knee, and lean in again. Work your way down to just above the knee—that usually feels wonderful because so many big muscles attach to the knee. Finally, lean the knuckles right into the middle of the top of your thigh and grind, just as you would with a mortar and pestle. Next, with the knuckles in the same spot, grind them forward and back, as if itching your thigh with your knuckles. Play with pressing harder with each of these moves to experience the different sensations you can make with your knuckles.

Grind and Glide

Place your knuckles at the top and center of the thigh, lean in, and use your body weight to press into your knuckles and glide them slowly to just above the knee. Try it on both the top and inside of the forearm, from wrist to just below the elbow. Using your knuckles makes your glides deeper.

Jiggling

Spread your hand wide across your thigh as if attempting to grab it, and with braced fingers and fingertips pressing into your thigh, jiggle your hand back and forth briskly. You'll feel the muscle sliding back and forth over the bone. Jiggling increases circulation and is a great way to wake up muscles and soften them while working on that area. I also use jiggling to cue a client that they're tensing an area—an arm, leg, or the head—and trying to hold it up when they should be relaxing into my hands. No helping allowed! A little jiggle prompts them to let that area go limp.

Kneading/Petrissage

Petrissage is a slow kneading motion, with both hands squeezing and squishing, pushing and pulling, like a cat. Cats make this movement as kittens while nursing, and this behavior seems to stay with them for life. When they knead your thigh into hamburger, it means "I love you." You've also seen or done this movement while kneading bread dough. Bread dough starts out cold and hard, and becomes soft and pliable as you knead. So do muscles; cold, tight tissue becomes warm and soft, and ready for deeper work.

Palpation

Palpating is an exploratory move. You can squeeze, rub, or gently press into an area just to feel the territory or locate the spot causing the trouble. Imagine you're feeling around in the muscle to find a marble in the tissue. Grab your upper forearm just below the elbow, and squeeze with your thumb and fingers. Smoosh the tissue over the bones. Press deeply here and there with your thumb. If you hit a tight spot that says, "right there," stop and hold that press. You've found a trigger point. Trigger points are common where the tendons attach at the top of the forearm near the elbow. Palpate your way down the length of the forearm, pressing your thumb firmly where it's most tender. Hold. Your forearm will thank you, and the other one will scream for equal attention.

Percussion

Percussion is repetitive thumping on a particular area. Percussion is great for really tight areas, such as the upper back and shoulders, to warm them up and increase circulation before doing deeper work. Put your hand in a "karate chop" position, and "chop" up and down your forearm a few times, as if it's bouncing along. With both hands, one after the other, chop the top of your thigh for a bit. When you stop, notice how tingly that area feels.

You can also use the sides of your fists for percussion on large areas, like the back and thighs. Make fists, and bounce them firmly and briskly up and down your thigh. Try it with all sides and angles of your fist, noticing how each position creates a different effect.

Pressing

Pressing on a tight area or knot coaxes that area to relax. You can press with your palm, heel of your hand, fist, thumb, or elbow, and the intensity of the press will increase in that order. The smaller the surface area, the more intense the sensation. You can press using the strength of your arms and shoulders; however, it's much easier on your own body and often more effective to lean your body weight into the press where possible, particularly the back and legs.

Press into the top of your thigh with your palm, then the heel of your hand, fist, thumb, and finally the elbow to experience the difference in intensity. Repeat each move, but this time, slowly rock your weight back and forth on each "tool." When pressing with the thumb, brace it and keep it in a straight line with the wrist. Don't let the thumb bend backwards at the bottom joint, as this creates a lot of stress on your thumb and will damage the joint over time. Brace your thumb in one long line from the wrist.

Rocking

Gently rocking the length of the body is another great way to begin or end a massage session. It's like "aloha"—it can mean hello *or* goodbye! We innately respond to rocking, right from birth. The movement is soothing and familiar, and we first experience it inside the womb, as our mother walks around. That's why rocking will calm even the fussiest baby.

Place both palms on either side of your thigh. Relax the whole leg. Push the thigh slowly back and forth, from one hand to the other. We don't want a jostle—just a very slow, gentle, rhythmic rocking, back and forth. Rock the thigh gently, as if you want to put it to sleep—then, just a slight bit more quickly, as if trying to gently wake it up.

Scratching

Gentle scratching is useful when working over clothing, and most people love it on the scalp. Scratch your forearm as slowly and lightly as possible, and continue scratching, gradually increasing the intensity, as if you're scratching a really pesky itch. Lightly drag your nails up and down the length of the forearm to create a totally different sensation. Scratching is actually quite versatile.

Gentle, firm scratching on the scalp melts most people into a puddle of *ahhhh*. Scratching over the sheet or clothing creates a gentle, light warmup for that area. Some people just absolutely love the sensation of fingernails slowly dragging over the skin, and if your loved one is amongst them, this is an easy technique to include in your Sacred Massage repertoire for almost anyone. Even moves that don't seem to have much therapeutic value may be pleasurable, which results in the release of calming hormones, which eases tension, and that *is* a therapeutic benefit after all!

Squeezing

Grab your wrist and squeeze, holding in this spot. Release and squeeze your way up the forearm to the elbow, and then release and squeeze your way back down. Play with the amount of pressure you put into the squeeze, from lightly to intense. Squeezing feels great on the arms and the tops of the shoulders, as well as the little muscles of the fingers.

You already squeezed the finger joints; now squeeze the muscles in between. The muscles of the fingers look like itty-bitty legs—squeeze those tiny thighs, calves, and soles to release tension in the fingers. Squeezing the knee also creates relief. Squeeze your knee, and move your hand into different positions, noticing how your knee appreciates this.

Smooshing

A smoosh is a squeeze that squishes everything as you're squeezing. Squeeze your forearm again, and hold. Now, work your fingers around that squeeze, as if softening a ball of hard clay in your hand. Smoosh your way up the forearm to just below the elbow, warming up and softening that hard clay.

Stripping

Just like stripping linoleum off a floor or ice off a windshield, you sometimes need a stiff, flat "tool" to strip away tension. You can strip with your knuckles or fingers braced together like a flat plane. Stripping is done along tendons or long strips of tight muscle, like along arms and legs. You aren't really stripping anything away, but rather, creating a deep, sliding friction that softens knots and tight areas, allowing the muscles and tendons to relax and move freely.

Brace your fingers into a flat plane, and on the inside of your forearm, place your fingers near the outer point of the elbow. Press deeply, and very slowly slide down the arm and over the wrist, stopping at the heel of the hand. To repeat, lift your fingers and start back at the top near the elbow. When stripping, you only go in one direction, the same way every time, not back and forth.

Try this same stripping motion with just your thumb. Grasp the forearm just under the elbow, and strip the thumb down to the heel of the hand. This creates a narrower "stripper" for smaller places. Because it's a smaller surface area, it's also more intense. Turn your arm over and squeeze it again, this time with the thumb on top of the forearm near the elbow. Find a trigger spot near the elbow and slowly strip down to the wrist. This move is great for those who spend a lot of time at a keyboard, playing musical instruments, or using hand tools.

Stroking

Stroking is basically a light one-way slide. Long, slow, strokes along the back, arms, legs, or face are very soothing and, like scratching, can be used to begin or finish working on any area, or the whole body. Stroking the hair is very calming, and another option for finishing up on the head or scalp. Gentle, slow stroking works well for those with fibromyalgia, on fragile, elderly skin, or on babies and infants. If soothing and calming is needed, gentle stroking can do the trick.

The Tools in Your Manual Toolbox

Your amazing hands can do almost anything, from performing microsurgery to painting a masterpiece to playing a piano concerto. Within the framework of massage, they're just as versatile. Each area of the hand, each position, can be used as a massage tool. The thumb can press. Your palms glide and slide. Your fingers can scrape and squeeze. Your fists can press an area flat or grind into a tight spot. Your knuckles can slide, scrape, and grind. The sides of your fists are great for percussion, and the heels of your hands allow you to lean your body weight into a tight spot and deepen pressure. Let's explore these manual "tools" one by one.

To simplify our conversation, rather than re-explaining the position and movement of your hands for each part of the body as we learn massage techniques, I've named each "tool" so you'll know immediately what I'm talking about. When I tell you to use your Duckbill or Steamroller, you'll know exactly what I mean. However, if you forget, no worries—tab this page so you can easily refer back to it if necessary. As you learn about these "manual tools," practice using them on various parts of your body to experience their usefulness, versatility, and depth.

Activity
GETTING TO KNOW YOUR TOOLS

Practice making each of the following tools, and say their names out loud as you do to help you remember them. Play with them a bit and see what sort of sensations you can make.

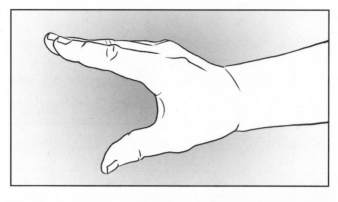

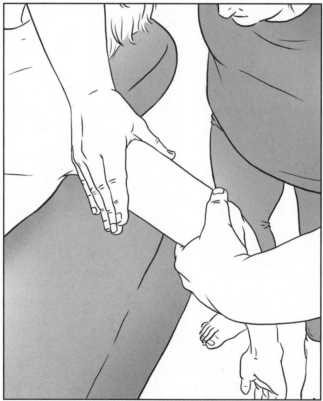

FIGURE 4: DUCKBILL MASSAGE TECHNIQUE

Duckbill

Straighten and brace your fingers into one plane, and straighten your thumb. Snap your thumb to your fingers. It looks like a duck's bill, right? Now, make the duck quack: *quack quack quack*. Use your Duckbill to squeeze an area, either holding firm in one spot or squeezing and sliding the area through the bill. Make a Duckbill, and squeeze your forearm and hold. Then pull your forearm through the bill to experience a deep, squeezy slide.

Iron

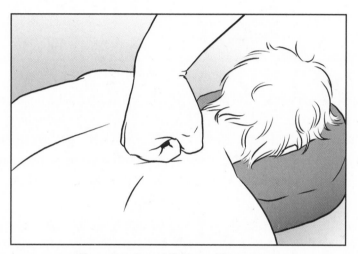

FIGURE 5: IRON MASSAGE TECHNIQUE

Your Iron is the flat of your fist—the surface between the row of knuckles at the base of the fingers and the middle row of knuckles. It's the part of the fist you'd use to punch something. Like a real iron, you slowly press across an area to smooth out the "wrinkles." You can make a soft Iron with a relaxed fist, and a firm one by squeezing your fist. Practice a soft Iron by leaning into your thigh, and press down to just above the knee, then practice a firm Iron the same way. A variation of this move is to use the middle knuckles, forming a wedge, which provides a more intense press. You can Iron just in one direction, over and over, or back and forth.

Paintbrush

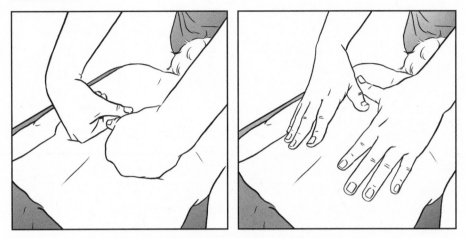

FIGURE 6: PAINTBRUSH MASSAGE TECHNIQUE

Your Paintbrush is a soft Iron on the way up, and soft, relaxed palm on the way back. Iron down the top of your thigh, and when you reach the knee, open your hand, palm down, and drag it all the way back to where you started. Your hand is relaxed and heavy in both directions, like a floppy wet washcloth, or big wet paintbrush. Imagine you are painting comfort with your hand, just like you'd paint a wall.

Powerpoint

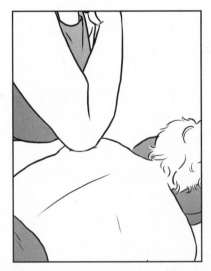

FIGURE 7: POWERPOINT MASSAGE TECHNIQUE

Your elbow is your Powerpoint, and you use it to press deeply into an area for a sustained bit of time. Use your Powerpoint if your thumbs are weak, or if you need more power than you can deliver with your thumbs, or just to give your thumbs a break. You can increase pressure with your Powerpoint with just your arm and shoulder strength; however, I find it more effective and easier to lean my chin into my palm, elbow bent, allowing me to make use of the strength in my upper back and shoulders as well as body weight. Powerpoints are great on trigger spots, or anywhere there's a thick, tight muscle that's hard to reach with your hands, such as deep in the glutes, or areas that are particularly rock-hard, like the upper back and shoulders.

Bend your elbow and place it in the center of the top of your thigh. Put your chin in your palm, and lean in, pushing with your upper back muscles. Experiment with the pressure. You'll discover that it doesn't take much to deliver a very intense, focused press. Practice leaning your Steamroller into your thigh until you learn to control your body weight and pressure very precisely. This tool should create a deep ache, but not a sharp, jabbing pain. A well-controlled Powerpoint on a trigger spot can definitely be uncomfortable, but not to the point of making someone tense up or pull away. They should be able to breathe through the discomfort, and if they can't, it's too deep. It should feel like leaning into a bruise, not like getting poked with a stick.

Rake

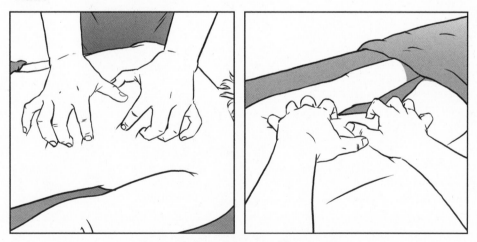

FIGURE 8: RAKE MASSAGE TECHNIQUE

Bend your hands into a halfway curve, like a growly bear with its paws up. *Grrrrr!* Brace your fingers in that position and rake the tops of your thighs, up and back. Experiment with both speed and pressure. Next, rake your hand along the top of the thigh only in one direction, starting at the knee and raking to pull toward you and then releasing to return to the knee and rake the thigh again. Add in the other hand, raking in one direction, one hand after the other. Raking is a great transition tool for moving from a slow, gliding warmup to deeper massage moves. It's wonderful on the back, sides, and calves.

Scraper

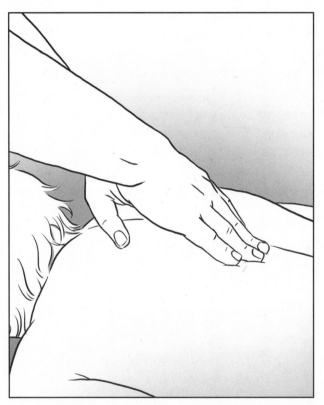

FIGURE 9: SCRAPER MASSAGE TECHNIQUE

Your straight, braced fingers, powered by your braced hand and straight, braced wrist, are your Scraper. Use your Scraper for stripping along muscles, and also across them, to loosen and soften long strips of tight muscles, tendons, and tight areas. You can do one long scrape, the length of the muscle, or press back and forth in smaller areas to increase circulation and soften. Place your Scraper at the top of the thigh, and scrape down to just above the knee. Pause there, and scrape briskly back and forth above the knee, just a few inches, all along the curve of the knee, noticing the muscle attachments there. Experiment with the pressure to find your preferred pressure along those attachments.

Snowplow

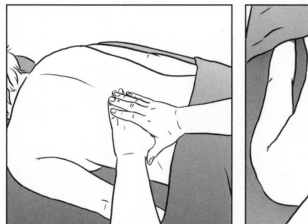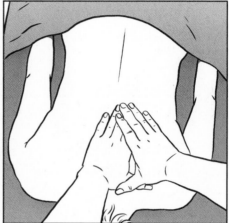

FIGURE 10: SNOWPLOW MASSAGE TECHNIQUE

This fun little tool gets its name from a skiing position for slowing down. You slide the back of your skis outward and the tips right next to each other, forming a wedge. In skiing, you lean into the backs of the skis in a Snowplow to slow down, and you do the same in massage. The movement, control, and pressure are driven from the heel of the hand, palm down, fingers extended. This creates a slow, deep, comforting slide.

To create your Snowplow, place one palm on your thigh, fingers straight. Put the other hand on top of it, with the fingers slightly angled so the middle fingers are near each other. The thumb of the top hand will rest right along the base of the other thumb, with the tip of the thumb touching the wrist. Lean onto your hands and slowly slide them forward, down to the knee. Release, return to your starting point, and slide again. You Snowplow in the same direction that your fingers point. The fingers point the way, and the heel of the hand provides the power.

Steamroller

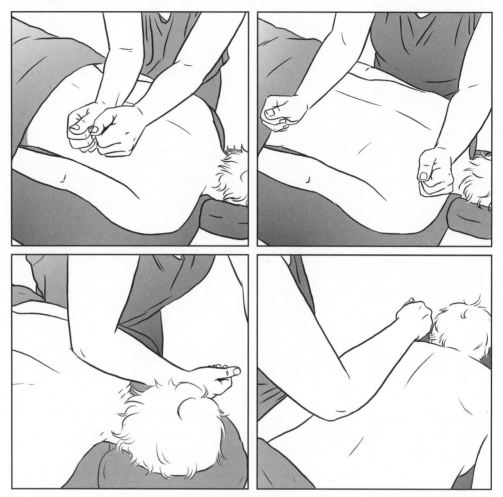

FIGURE 11: STEAMROLLER MASSAGE TECHNIQUE

Your Steamroller is your forearm, which you can use alone, or both arms together. Use your Steamroller to create a glide with deeper and longer or wider pressure. This move is great along the back and on the thighs.

Lean your forearm across your thigh, perpendicular, elbow to the outside of the thigh, hand draping on the inside of the thigh. Increase the weight of your lean to experience the pressure. Slide the forearm the length of the thigh to just above the knee. You can get the idea over clothing, but you'll experience this move more fully if you put on some shorts and use a little oil. This is a good way to practice controlling the speed of your glide while also applying pressure.

You can use one Steamroller alone to glide down the length of a long muscle, such as next to the spine, or you can use a double Steamroller by using both forearms at once by placing them together and then sliding them apart, in and out, across a large flat plane such as the back.

Practice, Practice, Practice

Some of the moves and tools we explored in this chapter may feel awkward at first, while others may feel perfectly natural. That's okay. It's all about the practice, and we're going to get plenty of that. Use your tools on your thigh or forearms whenever you get a chance, like while watching TV or waiting for the doctor to come in at your next appointment. Eventually, they'll feel as natural as if you'd been doing them forever.

Chapter 8

Touching the Back of the Body

We have arrived! We're finally ready to start learning and practicing the physical massage techniques of Soothing Touch! Now is when you'll need that massage table, and also that Body Buddy we discussed in chapter two. Going forward, you'll need both to learn the various techniques and sequences of massage.

We'll learn the sequences for each area of the body in the same order that I do them in a massage session: Back of the body first in this chapter, front of the body second in the next. That doesn't mean it's the only way to do it—it's just how I do it. You can swap things around and customize the sequences for your own preferences later on, but for the sake of learning and coherence, we'll learn everything in this particular order.

In both this chapter and the next, we'll assume that your Buddy is lying flat on a massage table: on their stomach in this chapter and on their back in the next. We'll also assume that your Buddy is covered with a massage sheet from shoulders to toes at all times, except when you are directed in the sequences to move the sheet. Before starting a practice session, direct your Buddy to remove all clothing and jewelry; underwear can stay on, however, because we'll learn and work that area over the massage sheet.

The table should be set near the top of your thigh, low enough to allow you to lean into the body when you need to increase pressure. Wherever possible, lower your own body by bending your knees rather than leaning over your practice partner, which reduces stress on your back.

When your Buddy is lying facedown, put a rolled towel, pillow, or bolster under their ankles to relieve pressure on the feet. Slide the support under the bottom massage sheet so it doesn't touch the skin. When faceup, the support can be placed under the knees beneath the bottom massage sheet to relieve pressure on the back.

Cheat Sheets

Beginning in this chapter, after each area and sequence, there are "cheat sheet" summaries for both specific areas and combined regions. Write them down in a spiral-bound or similar notebook as we go along. The process of writing them helps you memorize the sequence, but more importantly, you'll be creating a master set of cheat sheets for the full-body routine, which we'll be using later. There is also an appendix containing all of the cheat sheets in order. You can use either; however, if you make your own notebook, your book will stay much cleaner.

Your Buddy, Your Teacher

As you start practicing on your Buddy, you'll be asking more of them than to simply lie there and enjoy it. (Although that's part of the gig too!) Explain each practice session in advance: Where you'll be working, and what you'll be doing. Explain to your Buddy that they may experience a gentle, achy pain as you work on tight areas. That's not a bad thing. The right amount of pressure for relieving tight muscles, tendons, and ligaments should feel like a "delicious ache"—like pushing on a bruise. It simultaneously hurts and feels wonderful. Tell your Buddy that bruisy pain is great. Sharp pain, like a needle jab, is not.

If anything you're doing causes a sharp pain, or is so intense that your Buddy holds their breath, tightens that muscle to protect it, or feels the urge to pull away, it's too much pressure. Ask them to tell you immediately when it's too much so you can ease up or stop. Conversely, ask them to tell you when you hit the "Goldilocks" pressure: not too light, not too deep—just right.

Also, ask your Buddy to tell you when you hit a "sweet spot" so you can spend more time there. It's that spot makes you go, *"Ahhhhh"* and sigh, "More, more, more!" Remain on that spot, pressing or squeezing, and slowly increase the intensity to find that Goldilocks pressure. Most any muscle can have a sweet spot, particularly on the back, shoulders, neck, arms, legs, and glutes—the ones that do all the work.

Before beginning, ask your Buddy if they have any allergies (particularly to nuts), and check the ingredients in your oil or lotion. Ask if they have, or have had, any surgeries or injuries that might be aggravated by massage, or any chronic conditions such as arthritis or osteoporosis. If the answer is yes, avoid those concerning areas, and don't go any deeper than spreading oil over each area and exploring the structures under the skin very gently.

After the session, ask your Buddy for feedback: *What was great, and what was not so great? Is there anything I should do differently?* Feedback is invaluable for learning information, and your Buddy is your on-the-job teacher.

Let's Get Started

As we learn about each area, we'll focus on where various bones, joints, tendons, and muscles are and how they feel under your hands, rather than getting lost in the high weeds of memorizing human anatomy. (Whew, right?) When I was in massage school, our instructor told us, "For now, it's more important to know what's under the skin, what it looks like, and how to work on it than it is for you to remember its name." This approach worked well for me when I was starting out, so we'll do the same here. We'll take a kinesthetic approach, learning by doing, rather than by memorizing. Knowing the name of every body part won't make you an excellent massage therapist. But practice will. In fact, you could do a wonderful full-body massage without ever knowing the name of anything—but not if you weren't familiar with how a body feels and how to massage it. Massage isn't a verbal process—it's a kinesthetic one. You must know each part with your hands, not your brain. The more times your hands glide over an area, the more familiar it will become. It's like learning a dance—it's awkward now, but eventually you'll know all the steps by heart and it will be effortless.

Although we don't need to become fluent in human anatomy, we do need to learn a few anatomical terms so we can have a coherent conversation. If I were to say, "Press on the shoulder," you wouldn't know if I meant the top of the shoulder, the shoulder joint, or the upper back. But if I say, "Press on the trapezius," you'll know exactly what I mean. Let's learn a couple terms right now, because we'll be using these two a lot: "lateral" and "medial." "Lateral" means the side away from the spine, and "medial" means the side nearest the spine. This provides clarity, because if I told you to "put your hand on the outside of the calf," you might interpret "outside" as the skin, all over the calf. If I said the "inside of the calf," you might interpret that as right inside the muscle. Yuck! Gross!

Lateral   Medial

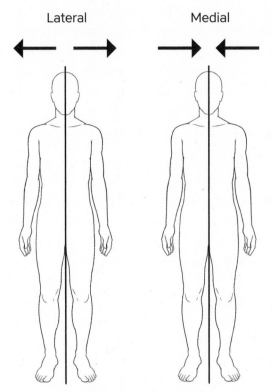

FIGURE 12: LATERAL VS. MEDIAL

Bottom line, don't stress too much about mastering the anatomical terms we'll be learn-ing. They'll come to you as we go along. And I promise—you won't need to pass an anat-omy test before I allow you to finish this book!

Study the Graphics

When you come to a graphic, look carefully at the picture—the shape, size and angle of the muscles, tendons, and bones—and trace the various muscles, bones, and tendons on your own body. Imagine the graphic under your own skin. Say the names out loud, and touch or flex that body part. By looking, tracing, and speaking each part, your brain gets three sources of input, which makes it easier to remember. When you practice on your Buddy, repeat this exercise. Open the book to the graphics, and visualize what's under the skin. Say the names out loud as you trace the bones, muscles, and tendons on your Buddy. If you forget the name of a certain body part, no worries—just return to the graphic.

Some of the pronunciations may look pretty hairy—go to the Google dictionary for the correct pronunciation if you wish. Besides pronunciations, you can also find plenty of supplemental information about anatomy online. There's no harm in learning more about anatomy if you're interested. In addition to consulting Dr. Google, there's plenty of free information at the library. Seek out illustrated, pictorial anatomy books, rather than books intended for medical training—the simpler, the better. A really fun way to learn anatomy is to get an anatomy coloring book. Crayons make everything happier!

How Does It Feel?

We'll learn about the body and its massage sequences like we did your "manual tools"— on your own body first, and then on your Buddy, with the exception of the upper back, which is nearly impossible to reach on yourself. We'll explore each area and sequence, part by part, step by step, until we know the steps for the whole dance: a full-body massage.

Learning to massage goes hand in hand (ha!) with becoming familiar with the body. How is it put together? How does each part feel? Where are the bones? What's between and over the bones? Where are the joints? Where are the tendons? Where do they connect? You've been living in your body your whole life, and I'll bet you don't know the answers to all of those questions! As we learn about the body, you'll be learning about your own body too.

Don't pressure yourself to plow through all the sequences full-speed. There's no pressure here, and it's not a competition. Take your time. Learn at your own pace. Learn one area, and when you feel confident about it, *then* move on to the next. Give your hands time to memorize how a body feels underneath them. You can repeat each sequence as many times as you like before moving on.

Same but Different

Although people come in all shapes and sizes, human anatomy is essentially the same on almost all people, but bodies may feel different from person to person depending on physical fitness, activity level, and body fat. The muscles of someone who sits on the couch all day will not look or feel the same as someone who lifts weights every day. They'll be the same muscles, but will differ in size, shape, and density. Imagine a ballerina's arm and a bodybuilder's—very different in appearance, but the very same muscles.

Skeletons are also essentially the same from person to person, with the exception of those who have congenital malformations, bone or joint disease, or severe skeletal injuries. However, bone density can vary. The bones of a healthy 20-year-old will be much denser than those of someone with osteoporosis. Babies' skeletons are different because some of the bones are still cartilage that will fuse together over time and become bone. A newborn's skeleton has more than 300 bones that grow and change over the years. By adulthood, there will be only 206 bones.

Body fat also makes one body feel different from another. The thicker the fat layer, the harder it will be to feel the muscles and bones, particularly on the back, upper arms, hips, butt, and thighs. But they're still there! As you feel for various soft tissue and bones underneath, be aware that fat layers can be very sensitive. Increase your pressure slowly to reach the muscles.

Speaking of Slowly...

With the exception of specific brisk moves intended to increase circulation, massage only has two speeds: slow and slower. Particularly when using oil, you must go very slowly until you learn to control the speed of your glide. You must be in control of your hands at all times, no matter how slippery the surface, so they don't go skating off where they shouldn't. Imagine you're feeling for a tiny marble hidden below that slick surface. Your touch must be firm and slow to find it. A slow pace also facilitates relaxation, whereas moving too quickly disrupts it. Rushing through the moves can generate anxiety and stress, rather than relieve it.

The Back

The back extends from the top of the shoulders to the top of the hips. However, the spine itself is much longer, beginning at the base of the skull and ending at the tailbone. The spine has four parts: the cervical (neck), thoracic (chest), lumbar (lower back), and sacral (below the hip line).

In spinal terms, your neck isn't separate from your back. It's all one long spine. The cervical spine runs from the base of the skull to the top of the shoulders and has seven vertebrae. The thoracic spine begins below the seventh cervical vertebra (which feels like a big bump on your back at about the shoulder line) and extends to just below the rib cage, and has twelve vertebrae. The lumbar spine begins where the thoracic ends, and has five vertebrae that end at the sacrum, a flat, wedge-shaped plane created by five fused vertebrae extending from the last lumbar vertebra to the tailbone. The sacrum is the back of the bones collectively called the "pelvic girdle." Protruding from the bottom of the sacrum is the tailbone, or coccyx.[65]

With the exception of the first cervical vertebra (which is ring-shaped and supports the skull) and the sacral vertebra, the vertebrae aren't round. They have bony protrusions called "processes" on the top and on each side. It's okay to press between the processes, but not directly into them. Never press directly onto the spine—always press just next to it, in the muscle tissue. Between each vertebra is a disc, which acts as a cushion, holds the vertebrae together, and allows for spinal movement and mobility.

The spinal cord is one long nerve running from the brain through the vertebrae of the entire spine, with nerves branching off into other parts of the body at each vertebra. These branching nerves can be pinched by bone, muscle, or cartilage, or a herniated spinal disc, resulting in tingling, pain, or numbness elsewhere in the body. A pinched lumbar nerve can radiate pain through the gluteus muscles and back of the thighs. A pinched cervical nerve can cause numbness, tingling, and pain in the arms and hands. If your loved one has limb numbness, tingling, or pain that doesn't have an obvious source, such as a pulled muscle, it may be from an impinged nerve. You can relax the muscle, but the source of the pain requires a visit to the doctor or chiropractor.

---

65. American Association of Neurological Surgeons, "Anatomy of the Spine and Peripheral Nervous System," AANS.org, accessed March 29, 2022, https://www.aans.org/en/Patients/Neurosurgical-Conditions-and-Treatments/Anatomy-of-the-Spine-and-Peripheral-Nervous-System.

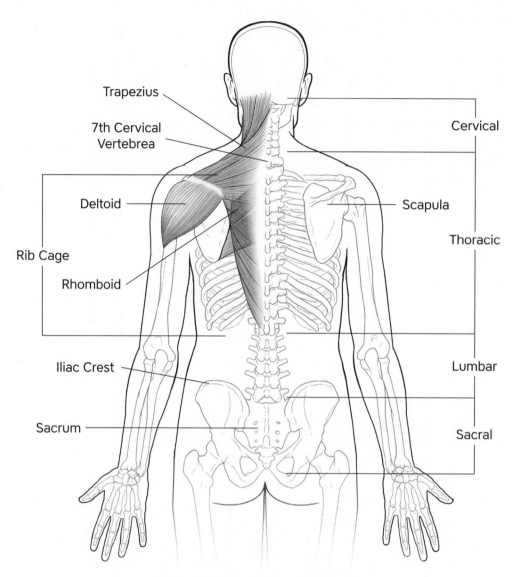

Trapezius

7th Cervical
Vertebrea

Deltoid

Rib Cage

Rhomboid

Iliac Crest

Sacrum

Cervical

Scapula

Thoracic

Lumbar

Sacral

FIGURE 13: BACK, SPINE, AND MUSCLES

On Yourself

It's very difficult to reach and feel your own back, particularly up between the shoulder blades, but there are still a few things you can self-explore.

Bend one arm behind your head, and place your fingers on your spine, as low as possible. Find the "bump" of the seventh cervical vertebra. Move your fingers over a bit, right between the neck and shoulder blade, and slide them down as far as you can. Brace and curl your fingers, dig in, and drag your curved fingers back up and over the top of your shoulder. Repeat with increasing intensity to experience that "delicious ache" in this notoriously tight spot. When you discover it, you may realize you need a massage yourself!

With your fingers, palpate and explore your rib cage, noting the difference between the bones and the muscle between them. Bend your elbow, place the heel of your hand as high up the side of your rib cage as you can, then press the heel of your hand down the side of your rib cage, noting where it stops and becomes soft tissue until you reach your hip bone.

Put your thumbs to the front of your stomach, and your fingers on your back, on the soft tissue between the rib cage and hips, in the lumbar area. Palpate, and see what you feel there. The triangular-shaped muscles in this spot hold your body erect, and allow you to twist and bend side to side. Your hands still in the same position, slowly bend side to side to feel these muscles working. You'll notice they move in opposite synchronization: When one side contracts, the other side releases. Bend forward and back to feel these muscles contracting and releasing together.

Slide your hands down further to your hip bones. They are the rounded upper corners of the ilium, a big curved, flat bone extending from the lower lumbar spine to the bones you sit on—often just called the "sit bones" (ischium, if you want to get fancy!). You have a matching ilium on each side of the sacrum, and together, they are the "ilia." The edge of the hip bone you can feel is the iliac crest, a "bony landmark" we'll be referring to frequently.

Sit down, place your hands on your sacrum, and press firmly. Wiggle around in your chair a little, and rotate your hips up and down, to see if you can detect the subtle movement of the sacrum.

On Your Buddy

Fold the sheet down to the tailbone. Without oil, run your palms all over the back, and just notice what you feel under your hands. Glide your hands in every direction, as if you were spreading baby powder over the skin. Notice the bumps and curves, the slopes and angles. Try to memorize *this* back with your hands—how it's shaped, how it's connected, how it feels.

Next, find the bony landmarks of the back:

Spine: With a fingertip, gently trace the entire length of the spine, from the base of the skull to the tailbone, identifying the four parts of the spine: cervical (base of the skull to the big bump at the base of the neck); thoracic (bump at the base of the neck to the bottom of rib cage) lumbar (bottom of rib cage to the top of the iliac crest); sacral (top of the iliac crest to the tailbone).

Scapula/Shoulder Blade: This flat, wedge-shaped bone lies on top of the upper rib cage, angling away from the spine from the top of the shoulder to below the armpit. Trace the outline of the scapula with a finger, imagining how it looks under the skin.

Rib Cage: Gently rake your fingers between the ribs from the spine to the side of the body. Notice that they aren't perpendicular to the spine—they slope slightly downwards from the spine. Find the bottom rib to locate the end of the rib cage.

Iliac Crest/Hip Bones: Trace the edge of the iliac crest, from the curve of the hip bone to the spine. You won't be able to feel much, if any, of the concave-shaped ilium itself because it's usually covered by the thick, deep muscles and fat.

Sacrum: One way to find the sacrum is to look for the two matching dimples in the lower back, which are located at the top of the sacroiliac joints. Trace the triangle formed by the dimples and the tailbone to locate the sacrum. There are muscles and ligaments attached to the sacrum, and nerves passing through it that can get pinched. Between the sacrum and each adjacent ilium are the sacroiliac joints, which can be a source of hip pain if inflamed.

Back Sequence

Before learning the actual massage techniques for the back, we'll begin with a gentle "rock and walk" to say "hello" to this body, and get it ready to be touched. Stand facing your Buddy's side, and put a palm on the point of each shoulder. Slowly and gently, rock the shoulders back and forth, as if rocking them from one palm into the other and back. Notice your Buddy's body rocking slightly with the movement.

Over the massage sheet, continue rocking your way down the body by walking your palms step-by-step down the rib cage, waistline, and hips; down the lateral sides of the thighs and calves (the side away from the spine); and on down to the feet. Give the feet a gentle, comforting squeeze. Slowly rock your way back to where you started.

Place the heels of both hands side by side on the upper back, between the scapula and base of the neck. The heels of your hands are next to the spine, not on it, your fingers draping softly over the spine. Rock your weight gently onto the heels of your hands, then rock back, and repeat. Again, your Buddy's body rocks along with your movement. When you feel ready, gently and slowly rock the heels of your hands down to the iliac crest, alongside the spine, then rock your way back to where you started. Do this a couple times until the rocking feels relaxed, natural, and familiar. Move to the other side and repeat.

Warming Up

Fold the massage sheet back to the tailbone, and spread some oil all over your Buddy's back with your relaxed palms—up and down, back and forth, and from corner to corner, practicing the control of your glide. Go *very* slowly. Think about the graphics of the bones and muscles of the back, and imagine your hands sliding over them. Slide over all the bony landmarks.

Move to stand facing the shoulder, angled toward the feet. Place your palms in Snowplow position at the top of the upper back, just below the shoulder, between the scapula and spine. Slowly, gently, firmly slide your Snowplow alongside the spine, walking alongside the body if necessary. When you reach the iliac crest, swoop up the "bunny slope" of the hips, make a U-turn, and slide back to where you started. Repeat until this feels comfortable and natural.

Practice deepening your Snowplow pressure by leaning a little body weight onto the heels of your hands as you slide. You must go slowly to control your glide. Ask your Buddy how this pressure feels. Do they want more, or is this enough? On your last plow, let your hand slide firmly down over the top of the shoulder, pressing in, which feels wonderful. Move to the other side of the body and repeat.

Return to your Snowplow starting position. With your hand that is closest to the body, make an Iron and place it on the upper back, just below the shoulder, between the scapula and spine. Iron just as you did your Snowplow—down the back next to the spine, to the iliac crest (the top edge of the hip bones on the back, above the glutes). When you Iron up the bunny slope of the hips and make your U-turn, switch hands and Iron with the hand that is now closest to the body, back to where you started. Repeat until this feels comfortable and natural, and once again, experiment with the pressure by leaning weight onto your Iron, checking in with your Buddy to see how this feels. Move to the other side of the body and repeat.

Stand facing the side of the body, angled toward the shoulders, and with your Rakes, rake over the shoulder and scapula, one hand after the other. Rake the rib cage, feeling the direction of the ribs. Rake over the soft tissue at the waistline, and stop at the iliac crest. Rake your way back to where you started. Move to the other side of the body, and repeat.

After these sequences, your Buddy's back should feel softer and warmer, and warmth may be building in your hands. Now, you're both ready to go a little deeper.

Going Deeper

Stand beside the shoulder, angled toward the feet. Bend the elbow of the arm closest to the head, and place your forearm at the top of the shoulder, between the scapula and spine. Now, you'll slide down the same track alongside the spine like you did during the warmup, but with your Steamroller. Lean into your forearm and steamroll down the back, but this time, when you reach the iliac crest, turn your Steamroller toward you and slide right off the lateral side of the body. Turn around, and place your other forearm parallel to the spine, elbow at the iliac crest, and slide back to where you started. Let your forearm slide all the way over the top of the shoulder, leaning in slightly as it goes over the top. You'll discover a natural groove right there on top of the shoulder, where your Steamroller easily slides on over. We'll call this the "Oh, *Yessssss* Groove."

Repeat until this feels comfortable and natural. Move to the other side of the body and repeat. As before, experiment with deepening the pressure by leaning in body weight, asking your Buddy to tell you when you achieve that "Goldilocks" pressure: deliciously achy. Be aware of your elbow at all times, making sure it isn't scraping against the spine.

Next, we'll use the Double Steamrollers. Stand facing the chest, and place your forearms right next to each other, across the middle of the back. Lean onto both forearms, staying on the muscle alongside the spine, not directly on the spine. Slowly slide your forearms apart, one toward the head, the other toward the hips. When you reach the head and the hips, slowly slide your forearms back together again to where you started. Repeat, repeat, repeat, and practice deepening your pressure. When this feels comfortable and natural, switch to the other side and repeat.

Let's give your "Powerpoint" a try next. Almost everyone seems to have a knot in the trapezius area of the upper back, which is a triangular plane of muscle formed by the scapula, spine, and top of the shoulder. Palpate the trapezius with your fingers until you find the knot—it may feel like a rope, or a little speed bump. Place your elbow on the knot, and just let it rest there. Lean onto your elbow slightly, as slowly as possible, concentrating on controlling your lean. Watch your Buddy's breathing, and as they exhale, lean in a little more. Ask your Buddy to tell you immediately if this is too intense, as well as to tell you when "that's enough." When you achieve the "that's enough" spot, pause and continue leaning in, without moving or adding any more pressure. Hold this position for a whole minute.

Lower Back Sequence

Stand facing the waistline, and place the palm of your hand nearest the hip onto the iliac crest, fingers facing the shoulders. Lean gently into the heel of the hand, and slowly slide it up to the bottom of the rib cage. Drag your palm back to where you started, and repeat.

Remaining in this soft area between the rib cage and iliac crest, slide the pads of your thumbs one after the other, from spine to the side, up and down alongside the spine. Recall how the triangular muscles of this area felt on your own back, and imagine you are softening and relaxing them with your thumbs. With your fingers in Scraper position, put your hands together in a wedge shape, and gently but firmly scrape up and down this soft lumbar area, back and forth, still recalling the feel of this area, still softening and relaxing.

Place your palm at the iliac crest, just as you started, and give a few slow slides to the lower back. On the last slide, continue up alongside the spine, and over the top of the shoulder.

Finish your practice on the back with nice, easy back-and-forth sliding with your palms, covering the entire surface of the back, and finally, slide your palms out over the shoulders.

Cheat Sheet
BACK

To help you remember the back sequence, write these steps in your notebook and place it where you can see it as you practice: rock and walk the body; glide and slide; Snowplow; Iron; Rake; Steamroller, one arm; Steamroller, two arms; Powerpoint on trapezius; palm slide on lower back; thumbs on lower back; Scraper on lower back; palm slide on lower back, ending at shoulder.

Shoulders and Scapula Sequence

Surely you've seen a massage ad where some blissed-out person is having their shoulders kneaded. That's the classic massage move everyone loves. Pain and tension in the shoulders and upper back are amongst the most common complaints. Study this graphic of the shoulders and scapula, noticing the angles of the muscles sweeping up from the spine, right over the scapulas. That big muscle on top is the trapezius, which forms a triangle from the spine to the top of the shoulder and up the back of the neck. It's a large muscle, and because the muscles of the shoulders and upper back are so interconnected, we'll learn about them together.

Four smaller muscles on the back of the shoulder (with names much too complicated for our purposes) make up what we commonly call the "rotator cuff," which stabilizes the shoulder, raises the arm over the head, and holds the humerus in place at the shoulder joint. Repetitive motion is the enemy of the rotator cuff, a common spot for strain and injury. A rotator cuff tear can be serious enough to require surgery. If your loved one has chronic shoulder pain and weakness, and cannot raise their arm much above parallel, this should be examined by a doctor. Avoid any deep work there until given the all-clear from a physician.

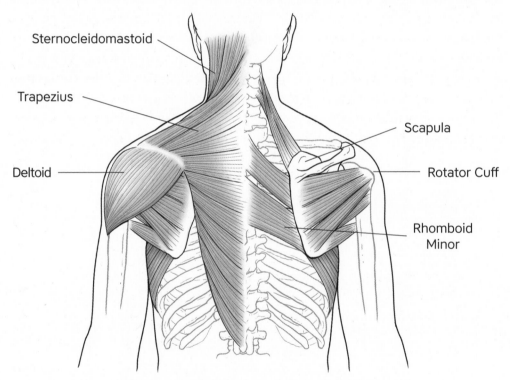

FIGURE 14: BACK OF SHOULDERS, SCAPULA AND NECK

On Yourself

You already explored as much as you can of your upper back, which is where the trapezius lives, so let's explore your shoulder a bit. Reach over your chest to your opposite shoulder. Rake your curved fingers all along the top of the shoulder. It may feel like a thick rope, and it may really appreciate your firm raking. Press your fingers firmly into that thick rope, and rotate your shoulder in both directions, then lift your shoulder up and down to feel this muscle move.

Before learning about the shoulder and scapula on your Buddy, let's make a Chicken Wing: Bend your elbow, bring your arm behind your back, and place the back of your hand on the small of your back, below the rib cage. In this position, the scapula lifts up a bit, allowing you access to the muscles running under the scapula. This is another "*Oh, yeaahhhh*" spot. Lots of muscle tension collects here. Notice how you must rotate your forearm a bit to take this position.

When you lift someone else's arm into this position, you must gently bend and rotate the elbow to place the hand on the back. While learning to make a Chicken Wing with someone else's arm, hold the forearm and hand, and ask them to place the back of their hand on their back, to see how the arm bends and moves.

On Your Buddy

Stand beside the rib cage, angled toward the head, and spread oil over the shoulders with both hands at once. Grab a shoulder in each hand, and do that classic massage move, squeezing and kneading, slowly and firmly. You can move your hands at the same time, or one after the other. Continue until the muscles feel nice and warm and squishy.

With both hands in Rake position, rake from the top of *one* shoulder down the trapezius to the bottom of the scapula, one hand after the other: When one hand reaches the bottom, it lifts and returns to the shoulder, while the other hand rakes down the trapezius. Keep repeating, one hand chasing the other. When this feels familiar and comfortable, move your Rakes to the other shoulder, and repeat. Notice how much more leverage you get while raking the shoulder across the body from where you're standing than you do while raking the one nearest you. Experiment with pulling deeper and deeper. The muscles of the shoulder and trapezius can take—and appreciate—deeper pressure.

Move to the other side of the body and repeat the whole sequence: knead both shoulders at once, then rake one shoulder at a time.

Now, it's time to make a Chicken Wing. Ask your Buddy to guide your hands as they rest the back of their palm on their lower back. Let the elbow flop. If it slides down the waist, that's okay. The scapula will still be lifted slightly. If this causes pain in the shoulder, abandon the Chicken Wing, and place the arm flat on the table alongside the torso. Even though the scapula won't be lifted, you can still do lots of good work in this area.

Trace the under edge of the scapula with your finger as you visualize the muscles and bones under the skin: the trapezius crossing over the upper edge of the scapula at an angle from the spine, and the rhomboids running underneath both the trapezius and scapula at the opposite angle. Palpate the area to feel the muscles and bones. That spot where the rhomboid dives under the scapula is a common trigger point, and a good place to experiment with your Powerpoint after the muscles are warmed up.

Stand beside the shoulder, facing the torso, and place your thumb at the bottom corner of the scapula nearest the spine, pressing in underneath until you feel resistance in the tissue. On some people, you can get your thumb pretty far under the scapula. On others, you can barely get under there at all. Either way, working this area feels wonderful.

With your fingers braced across the upper back near the trapezius, press your thumb up under the scapula, and pull your thumb toward your fingers, as if closing your hand. The fingers stay planted, and the thumb slides. Go slowly! Repeat until your Buddy feels that "delicious ache." You can place one hand on top of the other, and one thumb on top of the other, to brace your thumb and add more pressure by pushing with the top thumb into the bottom thumb. Keep practicing this thumb slide, experimenting with the pressure and checking in with your Body Buddy, until it feels comfortable and familiar.

Next, move to the top of the table to stand facing the shoulder. Brace your fingers on the trapezius again, and press and roll your thumbs—one after the other as if chasing each other—from the top of the shoulder, down the trapezius to the bottom of the scapula. Familiarize yourself with this area by playing with your other tools: Snowplow, Iron, Scraper, and Rake. Try them in both directions to see which you prefer. Practice sliding circles with your thumbs. When you're done exploring, go to the other side of the body and repeat each move.

Remember how we used the Steamroller in the back sequence? We'll use it just the same way to concentrate on the shoulder and trapezius. Stand beside the rib cage, angled toward the head. With the arm closest to the body, place your Steamroller parallel to the spine onto the trapezius, making sure your forearm is next to the spine, not on it.

Lean onto your Steamroller, and slowly drive it up the trapezius, then over the top of the shoulder. When you go over the top of the shoulder, lean into that "Oh, *Yessssss* Groove." Release, and drag your forearm over the upper arm, circling back to where you started. This is a great technique to practice controlling the lean of your weight and adding pressure, and checking in with your Buddy. Just remember: You *must* go slowly. When this feels comfortable and natural, move to the other side of the body and repeat.

If you're feeling saucy, you can also steamroll in the other direction: Face the shoulder, place your Steamroller at the top of the shoulder, drive it down the trapezius between the scapula and spine, release and circle the scapula with your forearm, drag it back to where you started, and repeat.

Cheat Sheet
SHOULDERS AND SCAPULA

To help you remember the shoulder and scapula sequence, write these steps in your notebook and place it where you can see it as you practice: knead both shoulders; Rake one shoulder with both hands, then the other; make a Chicken Wing; press thumb along under scapula; use tools of your choice on trapezius; Steamroll circles around scapula.

Neck

Most of the neck work is done while your Buddy is lying faceup, but the neck still gets a little attention while facedown. Remember that the trapezius and some underlying muscles stretch all the way up the back of the neck to the base of the skull. If your "traps" are tight, they're pulling all the way up your neck too. Shrug your shoulders as high and as hard as you can, and you'll feel your trapezius muscles contracting in your neck.

The neck's main job is to hold up your head, every day, all day. An adult head weighs ten to twelve pounds, which doesn't seem like a lot. But hold a ten-pound dumbbell out at your side, and you'll see how quickly it takes for ten pounds to feel like fifty. Imagine holding that dumbbell up all day, and you can appreciate how much work your neck does—while also moving and turning the head. No wonder so many people complain about stiff, tight necks!

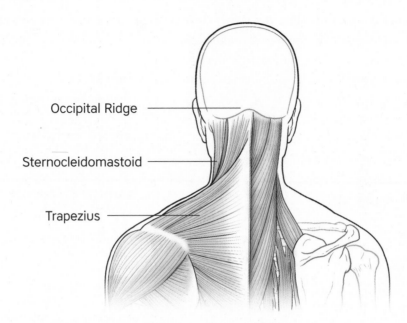

FIGURE 15: BACK OF NECK

Occipital Ridge

Sternocleidomastoid

Trapezius

On Yourself

Place your palm on the back of your neck, your thumb on one side and fingers on the other. Squeeze up and down the length of the neck, and notice how thick and tight these muscles are. Bend your neck side to side so you can feel the top of the trapezius working. Work your thumb and fingers in circles up and down the sides of the neck. If you're like most people, your neck may feel like one big "sweet spot" screaming for attention. Switch hands and explore the other side of your neck the same way.

Lie on your back, and lace your fingers behind your head, your thumbs on each side of your neck. Relax your neck, and press your thumbs firmly into the muscles on the sides of the neck, as if trying to push your thumbs together. Starting at the base of the skull, press your thumbs in small increments down the length of your neck to its base, and back up. Experiment with the pressure, noticing that these muscles can take—and enjoy—very deep pressure.

Sit up, tilt your head to the side, and relax your neck, letting your head hang over the shoulder. Cross the arm on that same side over your chest, and palpate the length of the trapezius, from the shoulder to the skull. With your Rake, pull from back to front along this long plane of muscle. Place your palm on the side of your head, and gently pull toward the shoulder, feeling the stretch in the neck.

With Your Buddy

Stand facing the neck. Grasp the neck in your Duckbill, thumb on one side of the neck, fingers on the other. Palpate. Feel the bones, muscles, and tight spots. Squeeze and knead with your Duckbill. Slide your Duckbill up and down along the length of the neck, feeling those tight muscles. When this feels comfortable and natural, move to the other side of the body and repeat.

Stand above your Buddy's head, facing the feet, and place one heel of each hand midway up the sides of the neck. Firmly slide the heels of both hands at once down the sides of the neck and out over each shoulder, along the same long strip of muscle you stretched with your head tilted. Repeat several times, going one way only—neck to shoulder—and increase the pressure by leaning into your hands. Repeat the same move using your Irons.

Finish by giving the scalp a nice, gentle scratch.

Cheat Sheet
BACK OF THE NECK

To help you remember the sequence for the back of the neck, write these steps in your notebook and place it where you can see it as you practice: Duckbill the neck; knead, squeeze, and slide; repeat on other side; slide heels of hands from neck to shoulder; slide Irons from neck to shoulder; gentle scalp scratch.

All Together Now: Back/Shoulders/Neck

Because the muscles of the back, shoulders, and neck work in concert, you'll flow right from the back sequence into the shoulders, scapulae, and neck. As these sequences become familiar, you can customize the order in which you prefer to do these moves or sequences. In general, warm and soften each area before going deeper. Play with the tools and techniques, and discover how they work better for some areas and not for others. Add in the ones you like, discard the ones you don't. As long as it works, and your Buddy likes what you're doing, it's all good.

Practice the sequences for the back, shoulders, and neck all together as one sequence for the back of the upper body. When you're done with the complete upper body sequence, finish by standing at the head of the table, facing the feet. Slide both palms simultaneously down each side of the back to the hips, then swoop them outwards to circle over the hips, and reconnect on each side of the spine.

Drag your relaxed palms slowly up the back like heavy, wet washcloths. At the top of the back, swoop your palms outward over each scapula, just like you did the hips, circle over the upper arm, and reconnect your palms on each side of the spine. Swoop back down to the hips, and repeat until this feels like one long, easy, relaxing sequence. It's sort of a big "doggy bone" pattern. On the last pass, swipe your palms up the back of the neck, then press down the top of each shoulder simultaneously, finishing with one palm on the point of each shoulder. Pull the massage sheet up to cover the back. The "cheat sheet" for the back of the upper body is the cheat sheets you already wrote for the back, shoulders, and neck, combined.

Foot (Sole)

We'll begin learning about the back of the lower body at the feet. Some foot work is done while your Buddy is facedown, and a bit more when they're faceup. Like the neck, the feet work very hard, every day. They balance all our weight and absorb impact with each step, often while constrained in unnatural positions by cute but tortuous shoes. Those who are on their feet all day, or who run or participate in sports, are giving their feet a daily beating. We often don't realize how much chronic pain we're holding in our feet until a massage therapist starts pressing into them.

The soles of the feet are full of nerve endings and layers of muscles and tendons, and can be very tender and sensitive. Many people twitch or giggle when their soles are touched, and may need a little desensitization first. Place your relaxed palm firmly against the sole of the foot until the area calms down. Coach your Buddy to focus on breathing deeply and relaxing their foot.

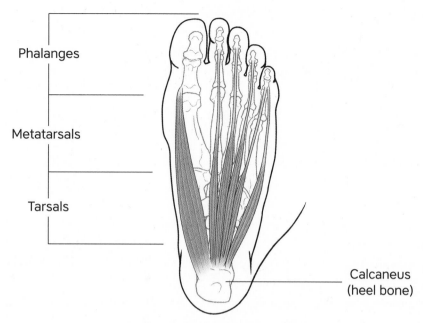

Phalanges

Metatarsals

Tarsals

Calcaneus
(heel bone)

FIGURE 16: BOTTOM OF FOOT/SOLE

On Yourself

Sit on a chair or the floor and pull one foot up onto the opposite thigh or knee. Grab the foot, fingers on top, thumbs on the sole. Press into the sole, exploring the sensations. Press into the ball, into the arch, and just below the heel. Rotate the foot with both hands, noticing how mobile the bones are. Place your knuckles across the foot, just below the heel, and push them down the sole to the ball and back, in a slow scrubbing motion. Massage the arch with your thumbs, pushing in deep slow circles.

Grab each toe at its base, and slowly, firmly slide up the length of the toe, feeling the toes stretch. You may even hear a pop in the joints like when you crack your knuckles. This harmless sound is made by dissolved gases expanding in the synovial fluid in the capsule between the bones,[66] and is commonly heard in the fingers, as well as neck and back when adjusted by a chiropractor.

---

66. Scientific American editors, "What Makes the Sound When We Crack Our Knuckles?" *Scientific American*, last updated October 26, 2001, https://www.scientificamerican.com/article/what-makes-the-sound-when/.

With your index finger, bend each toe down toward the sole, one at a time, then press backwards toward the top of the foot. Run your fingers through the toes, stretching them apart sideways. Grasping all the toes at once, press them all toward the sole, feeling the stretch in the top of the foot. Press them backwards toward the top of the foot, and push your heel down to feel the stretch in the sole and Achilles tendon.

On Your Buddy

Leave the support under the ankles, and fold back the massage sheet to uncover one foot. Spread oil over the sole, and place your Iron just below the heel bone. Press slowly down the sole to the ball. Return to the heel and repeat, heel to ball, in one direction. Make slow, firm circles with your Iron all over the arch.

Take the foot in both hands and lace your fingers underneath, your thumbs on the sole. Slide slow, deep thumb circles all over the sole. Give extra attention to the arch, as well as the bony point at the bottom of the heel bone. This point is where plantar fasciitis—a very painful inflammation of the fibrous tissue (plantar fascia)—causes so much grief. Press deeply on and below that point with your thumbs, up and down, then crossways like scissors.

Place both palms on either side of the heel, clasp your fingers, and squeeze your hands together as if trying to squish the heel in your palms. Squeeze your clasped hands in circles over the heel bone a few times.

To finish, run your palm down the sole, heel to ball, and drag your fingers gently through the toes.

Cover this foot with the sheet, and fold it back to expose the other. Repeat the entire process on the other side, ending with both feet covered by the sheet.

Cheat Sheet
FOOT (BOTTOM)

To help you remember the sequence for the feet while facedown, write these steps in your notebook and place it where you can see it as you practice: Iron sole; Iron circles on sole; thumb circles on sole; squeeze and squish heel; brush sole and toes.

Legs: Push Toward the Heart

As we move toward working on the legs (back and front), aiding circulation is one of the goals. The heart pumps blood away through the arterial system on the way out, and the blood is returned through the veins. We want to assist the heart in its job, so when working on the legs, particularly long, sweeping strokes, apply pressure as you move toward the heart, and release it on the way back. You can lift your hands and start your slide over where you began, or drag or glide them back to that starting point and repeat.

Calf

We think of the calf as one big muscle, but it actually has two major muscles. The big one, which gives the calf its shape, is the "gastrocnemius" ("gastroc" for short). This muscle has two bulbous "heads" on each side. When we talk about the calf, we're usually talking about the gastroc. Immediately underneath the gastroc is the soleus, a wide, flat muscle that extends from the back of the knee to under the Achilles tendon, which is actually much longer than just the visible tendon we can see and feel. This tendon attaches to the back of the heel bone, and then flattens and widens as it extends up to the bottom of the gastroc. It is the thickest tendon in the body, and anchors the gastroc and soleus to the heel bone.

These three structures in the calf make it possible to run, walk, and dance, and they get a lot of use and wear and tear, just living everyday life. If your loved one is an athlete, particularly a runner, their calves may get tight and sore, and deeper work may be a relief. However, you must be particularly careful when going deeper on the calf, because although the gastroc is big and strong, it's also amazingly tender. If you drive your Steamroller or Iron into the muscle without warming it up first, it will create a shock of pain in the calf. Ease into deeper calf work slowly, and in increments.

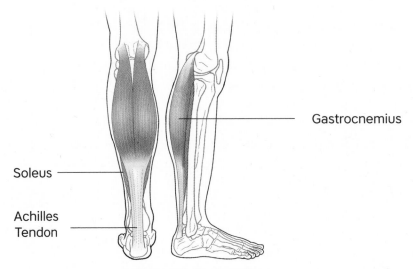

Gastrocnemius

Soleus

Achilles
Tendon

FIGURE 17: BACK OF CALF

On Yourself

Sit in a chair, with your soles flat on the floor. Grab one calf with your hand, fingers on the outside of the leg and thumb on the inside. Relax your calf, grasp it firmly, and jiggle it around. It will slide easily over the bone. Still grasping the calf, push up and down into your toes, flexing and pointing, to feel the gastroc moving. Slide your hand below the gastroc to the soleus, and flex and point again to feel this muscle move.

Press the flat of your "Iron" into the top of your gastroc, and press to slide downwards, stopping above the visible part of the Achilles tendon. Notice how tender the soleus is just above the Achilles tendon.

On Your Buddy

With a support under the ankles, fold the massage sheet back to expose one calf, tucking it between the legs. Face the side of the calf, and spread oil and palpate. Find both "heads" of the gastroc, the soleus, and the Achilles tendon.

Grasp the calf in both hands, and jiggle the muscle to warm it up. Ask your Buddy to relax their calf and just let it jiggle. To warm up the calf, knead the muscle with both hands, pressing and squeezing, one hand at a time, like a cat.

When the muscle is warmed up, place the heel of your hand at the bottom of the lateral (away from spine) side of the gastroc, lean in slightly, and slide your palm slowly and firmly up over that lateral head. At the top, let your palm slide off the lateral side, lift up your hand, and return to where you started, sliding only in one direction. Repeat a few times, then do the same slide on the medial (closest to spine) side of the gastroc, sliding off toward the medial side at the top. Stay with this move and repeat, experimenting with adding pressure and checking in with your Buddy. (You sometimes get instant feedback, because too much pressure on the calf can make a person yelp.)

Repeat this move—sliding up and off each side of the gastroc, but this time, use your Iron. Once again, experiment with the pressure and ask your Buddy to tell you when "that's enough."

Another way to deepen this move is to use your Steamroller. Stand angled toward the head, and place the forearm of the arm closest to your Buddy at the base of the gastroc. Angle your forearm so your hand drapes down over the lateral side. You will apply pressure with your forearm only, not the elbow. Lean into your forearm, and slowly slide it up and over the lateral-head gastroc, slide outwards at the top just as before, and lift your forearm to return to your starting point. To steamroll the medial side, keep your forearm at the same angle, but slide it so your elbow is further away from the calf. Slowly slide up and over the medial head of the gastroc, slide off the medial side, lift, and return to start.

Grasp both sides of the gastroc, one in each hand, right in the bulgiest part. Slowly squeeze and knead each side firmly, one hand after the other, like you're softening big balls of cold bread dough.

Slide one hand down the soleus to the Achilles tendon, and carefully grasp the tendon in your Duckbill. Do some slow, firm slides up and down to soothe the Achilles tendon.

To finish, slide your palms up the length of the calf and back down, over the Achilles tendon, over the heel, and down the sole. Gently brush your fingers over the toes. Cover the leg with the massage sheet, and repeat the entire sequence on the other calf.

Cheat Sheet
CALF

To help you remember the sequence for the calf, write these steps in your notebook and place it where you can see it as you practice: jiggle and knead; palm slides on both sides of gastroc; Iron on both sides; Steamroll both sides; knead both heads of gastroc at once; Duckbill slides on Achilles tendon; palm slides up and then down all the way over sole.

Thigh

The thighs contain some of the longest, largest muscles in the body, and most have more complicated names than we want or need to know. These muscles move, power, or stabilize the leg in different ways and directions. The common name for that big bulging muscle on the back of the thigh is the "hamstring," and for our purposes, that will do.

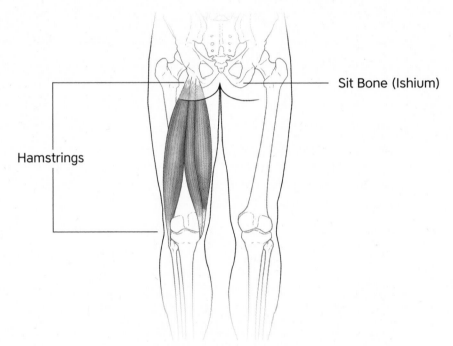

FIGURE 18: BACK OF THIGH

On Yourself

Put one foot up on a chair, knee bent, and relax the back of your thigh. Grab the muscle and jiggle it and let it flop, just as you did with your calf. Palpate to find the hard, ropy tendons attached to the back of the knee. Slide your hand back to just below your butt, and probe around to feel the attachments there, near the "sit bone." Slide your palm all over the back of your thigh to feel the surface. Unless you're fairly thin and fit, it's hard to distinguish one muscle from the next on the back of the thigh, and it will feel pretty much like one big muscle.

On Your Buddy

Fold the massage sheet up to just under the butt on one leg, and tuck it between the legs, leaving the entire back of the leg exposed. Without oil, explore and palpate the back of the thigh, and the tendons and attachments. Facing the side of the thigh, grab that big thigh muscle in the bulgiest part with both hands, and jiggle it. Place the heels of your hands on the lateral side of the thigh, and rock your weight back and forth into your hands to feel the movement of the muscle over the bone. Notice how the leg moves loosely and easily at the hip joint as you rock the thigh. Spread some oil over the thigh, kneading, softening, and warming.

Place your palm just above the knee, and lean in to push and slide the palm up the center of the thigh, swooping off the lateral side at the top, just below the butt. Release, return your palm to start, and repeat. Experiment with leaning in weight to increase the pressure. Like the upper back, the back of the thighs can take a lot of pressure. Angle your hands a bit each time so you cover the surface of the back of the thigh with palm slides.

Repeat this same move, using your Iron, and once again, experiment with the pressure and angle until you've Ironed the whole surface. Repeat again with your Steamroller: Angle your body slightly toward the head, and with the arm closest to your Buddy, place your elbow just above the knee on the inner (medial) side, your forearm angled so your hand drapes over the lateral side of the thigh. Lean in weight to slide your Steamroller up the back of the thigh, sliding off to the lateral side just below the butt. Lift your arm, return to start, and repeat. Experiment with adding pressure, and get feedback from your Buddy.

Wrap it up with a little more kneading and some palm slides, and on the last slide, at the sole, finish by sweeping your palms up over the calf to the top of the thigh, and back down the whole leg again, and over the heel and sole in one smooth move, gently brushing over the toes.

Cover the leg with the massage sheet, and repeat the entire sequence on the other side.

Cheat Sheet
THIGH (BACK)

To help you remember the sequence for the back of the thigh, write these steps in your notebook and place it where you can see it as you practice: jiggle and rock; knead, soften, and warm; palm slides; Iron; Steamroll; knead and slide; sweep over entire leg.

Glutes

Oh, our poor aching glutes! The gluteus maximus—our "butt cheek"—is the largest muscle in the body. It does much more than serve as a convenient cushion to sit on. It stabilizes the hips and torso for erect posture, and assists the thigh to move in any direction, including lifting it up.

The three gluteal muscles attach to the ilium. At the deepest layer is the gluteus minimus, lying directly at the top of the ilium and extending to the "greater trochanter," which is that big knobby bone at the top of the lateral side of the thigh. The fan-shaped gluteus medius is layered over the minimus, and also attaches to the ilium at the top and the greater trochanter at the bottom. The gluteus maximus is the large, round muscle on the top that we can see—the one that looks good in tight jeans. The gluteus maximus angles out from the sacrum and medial iliac crest to attach to the upper lateral femur (thigh bone).

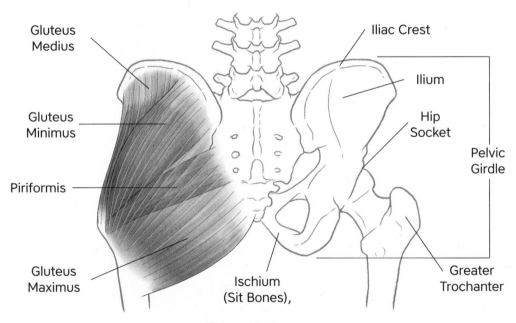

FIGURE 19: GLUTES

The gluteus maximus is big and thick, and protects the medius and minimus—so well that we may not realize the underlying muscles are sore until someone starts poking around there. These muscles work very hard, but we adapt to discomfort there, tuning it out like background noise. Your Buddy may be a little startled by how tender the glutes are, so approach work on this area slowly.

There are lots of other muscles in the butt, with lots of fancy names, but we really only need to know one more: the piriformis. You can just call it "The Spot," because when you press into the glutes and hit it, your Buddy may go *"Gaaahhh,"* in combined pain and relief. Pressing deeply and holding on the piriformis helps to relieve tension in the glutes.

Unless I'm doing very deep, concentrated work, I work the glutes area over the sheet, not for any particular reason other than that's how I learned to do it. As a non-professional, working the glutes over the sheet is more appropriate when massaging your loved one, and helps them feel safely and securely covered in this area. In addition, there are some bonuses for working the glutes over the sheet. It provides some traction, which actually comes in handy for doing deeper moves on the glutes. Nothing slides, and you can press in to slide the muscle over the bone, rather than your hands sliding over the surface. To get an idea of what that feels like, press your Iron against your cheek (the one on your face!) and make big circles, feeling the cheek slide easily over the bone. This is what you want to do with the other set of cheeks too.

On Yourself

Stand up and grab your butt with both hands, and press your fingers into the muscle. Walk around a bit, do some knee-bends, and lift your thighs in front of you, then to the back, and to the side, noting how the muscles move for each movement and position.

Find your greater trochanter, and press your hand in a semi-circle around it. You'll find a big curved gutter formed by the greater trochanter and the bottom of the ilium, traveling right over the hip socket. This gutter is a great workspace for the glutes. To feel your greater trochanter, press your palm over it and swing your leg in front of you to the opposite side of your body. You'll feel it pop out a little, and go back in place when you swing the leg back.

It's a little difficult to find your own piriformis, but you can try. Probe the center of your glutes with stiffened fingers. Pressing into The Spot often creates a slight burning sensation.

On Your Buddy

Because we'll work the glutes over the massage sheet, underwear can stay on—or come off. It doesn't really matter either way. Go into these moves very slowly, and carefully control your body weight when increasing pressure.

Face the hip. Press the heels of both hands into the heart of the gluteus maximus, and rock back and forth into the muscle as you did with the thighs. Notice how deep the muscle really is. With the heels of your hands or your Scrapers, palpate to find the curved gutter formed by the greater trochanter and lower ilium, and use your Iron to travel back and forth along that gutter, pressing in to slide the muscle over the bone.

Place both Irons side by side on the center of the glutes, and lean in to slide the muscle in circles over the bone, first one way, then the other. Imagine the big bowl shape of the ilium, and pretend you're wiping the sides of that bowl with the muscle. Remember, you are pressing into the sheet to create traction for moving the skin and muscle underneath—not sliding the sheet over the skin.

Walk your Irons all over the glute, slowly and deeply, as if punching into a ball of deep, cold dough. Keep walking and warm the dough up.

Next, we'll search for the piriformis. Anchor and brace the fingers of both hands near the sacrum, and place one thumb over the other to provide more leverage. Use the braced thumbs as one unit to slowly and deeply press into the glutes until your Buddy says, "That's enough." Move your thumbs a bit and repeat, until your Buddy says, "Oh, wow! That's really sore." Or maybe just yelps. Congratulations—you found The Spot! Stay there and hold for one minute.

Repeat with your Powerpoint: Slowly lean your elbow into The Spot, very lightly at first, leaning in more weight ever so slowly, until your Buddy says, "Enough." Hold for one minute. I find that I can deepen my Powerpoint more efficiently by leaning my chin onto my fist like "The Thinker" statue and pressing with my head too. You must lean in slowly because the piriformis can be an extremely tender trigger point. Don't just shove your elbow in there full-force, without warning, or you may get kicked in the face!

Leaning into the piriformis is a perfect opportunity to practice using your Powerpoint, which is great for other trigger points too, such as the rhomboids, the trapezius, the strips of muscle alongside the spine, and on top of the shoulders, on those troublesome "knots." Use your Powerpoint on soft tissue only, never on bone or joints. Practicing on the glutes over the sheet takes away the slippage factor, making it easier to learn how to control your speed and depth while leaning in body weight: the slower, the better.

To finish up this area, walk your Irons all over the glutes just like you did when you began.

Cheat Sheet
GLUTES

———

To help you remember the sequence for the glutes, write these steps in your notebook and place it where you can see it as you practice: rock glutes with heels of hands; Iron curved gutter between lower ilium and greater trochanter; Iron glutes with both hands to "wipe the bowl"; walk Irons to "punch the dough"; press and hold thumb on The Spot; lean Powerpoint into The Spot; walk Irons over glutes.

All Together Now:
Feet, Calves, Thighs, Glutes

While exploring the feet, calves, thighs, and glutes, we learned one area at a time: first one side, then the other. Just as we did with the upper body, we'll now combine all four areas into one lower-body region, doing the back of one entire leg and glutes, then the back of the other. Repeat each sequence in order—foot, calf, thigh, glutes—then repeat on the other leg.

When folding the sheet back to work the whole leg, just fold it back to expose where you need to work, tucking it between the legs, until the whole back of the leg is finally exposed. Cover the leg back up to proceed to the glutes. Finish the entire back of the leg as you finished the thigh—sweep your palms up from the sole to just under the butt, and sweep back down, brushing over the toes.

The cheat sheet for the entire back of the leg and glutes is all of the cheat sheets for these areas combined.

From Back to Front

Congratulations! You've just finished the basic massage sequences for the back of the body! In the next chapter, we'll flip over to the front of the body. Following that, we'll connect everything into one flowing full-body Soothing Touch routine. Once we're familiar with the full-body sequence, we'll plug it right into the overall Sacred Massage template, in one big, flowing, divinely magical experience.

And by the way—if you're wondering—yes, you *can*!

Chapter 9

Touching the Front of the Body

Just as in the last chapter, as we transition to the front of the body to learn more Soothing Touch techniques, we'll assume that your Buddy is lying faceup on a massage table, covered in a massage sheet from collarbone to toes, with a bolster, pillow, or support under the bottom sheet beneath the knees. We'll follow my own sequence for learning the front of the body, which you can customize later on.

Once again, I'll mention anatomical terms only as necessary for clarity and coherence. Knowing how each area feels, knowing what's where, and knowing how to work on that area take priority over memorizing names. As in the last chapter, study the graphics so you understand what's underneath the skin and how it's all connected, and recall those images as you practice on your Buddy.

The Flip Side

It's time for the part of a massage that everyone dislikes most: turning over. At this point of relaxation saturation, turning over feels like an unreasonable demand. But, until someone makes a pancake flipper for people, turn over we must.

After finishing the back side of the body, slide one arm under the feet and lift gently, while removing the support under the feet with the other. Stand facing the waist, and pin the sheet to the side of the table snugly with your thighs so it can't slide. With the hand nearest the shoulder, reach across the body and grab the top edge of the sheet. With the other, reach across the body and grab the sheet near the hip. Lift both arms at once in a V-angle, forming a little tent under which your Buddy can turn over. Ask them to scoot down the table, out of the face cradle, so they're lying completely on the table. The top of the head should not be over the edge of the table. Place the sheet back down over them, covering from collarbone to toes. Fold the top of the sheet over if it's too high. Remove the face cradle and set it aside.

People are often all askew after turning over. If your Buddy is at a diagonal or too near the edge of the table, pick up both feet under the heels, place them in the middle of the bottom of the table, and tell them to wiggle and scoot their hips and shoulders a bit until their body is aligned with their feet. Smooth all the wrinkles from the top massage sheet.

Slide one arm under the bottom sheet beneath the knees and lift. With the other, slide the support under the sheet and knees. Propping the knees releases stress on the lower back in this position. As with the back of the body, do each move slowly, and check in with your Buddy about the pressure. We'll begin where we left off: at the feet.

Foot (Top)

You probably already know there are five long bones in the foot, called metatarsals, each running from the upper foot to the ball, where there's a joint for each toe. The toes each have three smaller bones, called "phalanges," with the exception of the big toe, which has only two. At the other end of the metatarsals is a cluster of chunky bones, just in front of the heel. These are the "tarsals."

All together, there are twenty-six bones in the foot—there's one for your next trivia contest! But wait, there's more! The foot also has thirty joints and more than one hundred muscles! The foot is actually a rather complicated structure, and takes the impact of every step you take over the course of your life. The feet take an incredible pounding on a daily basis, and deserve some love. Like a couple other overused parts of the body, we often don't realize how sore our feet are until someone starts massaging them.

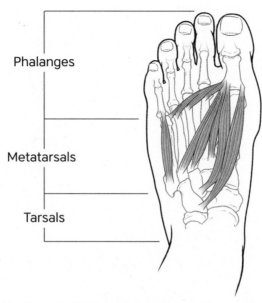

FIGURE 20: TOP OF FOOT

On Yourself

Prop one foot up on your knee, and palpate the top to find the tarsals, metatarsals, and ball, and the joints and bones in the toes. The tarsals may feel like one lump of bone. Grab each side of the foot, twisting and bending it in every direction, to experience the bones and joints flexing together. Press your thumb and forefinger between each metatarsal, and glide down between the bones to feel the soft tissue in between.

On Your Buddy

Standing at the foot of the table, fold the sheet back to expose one foot. Without oil, palpate the foot to locate the bones and soft tissue between them. Press your thumb between each metatarsal, and glide down to the ball, continuing all the way between the toes. Press along the phalanges of each toe, then grasp the toe pad and gently pull just to the point of resistance. Slide your fingers between the toes to gently stretch them apart.

Spread some oil over both sides of the feet. Now, we'll go double Duckbill: grab the foot in both hands at the top of the tarsals, thumbs on top of the foot, fingers on the sole. Slowly and firmly squeeze your Duckbills, as if pulling thick toothpaste from the tarsals to the toes. Do this several times, and feel the foot warm and soften. Grasp the foot firmly, moving your hands in alternate circles, as if loosening the bones in a figure eight. Go in both directions. Squeeze out the toothpaste with your Duckbills again.

Brace the foot in one hand, and with the knuckles of the other, grind them up and down the sole of the foot. Use your thumbs to press and slide over the arch a few times.

Slide your palm down the top of the foot to the toes, and gently press on the toes to curl them toward the sole, giving the top of the foot a nice stretch. Grasp the heel with one hand to stabilize the foot, and place the other palm underneath, on the ball. Simultaneously pull on the heel while pushing the ball upward toward the top of the foot, gently stretching the Achilles tendon. Squeeze out some more toothpaste with your Duckbills, and on the last squeeze, brush your fingers over the toes.

Cover the foot with the sheet, and repeat on the other side.

Cheat Sheet
Foot (Top)

To help you remember the sequence for the foot while faceup, write these steps in your notebook and place it where you can see it as you practice: double Duckbill toothpaste squeeze; loosen foot in figure eight; more toothpaste squeezes; knuckle grind sole; thumb presses on arch; slide down foot over toes, press toes toward sole, stretch top of foot; press ball toward top of foot while pulling on heel, stretch Achilles tendon; more double Duckbill squeezes; brush over toes.

Lower Leg

When working the front of the lower leg, between the ankle and knee, you're concentrating on the muscles alongside the shin, which include the front portions of the gastroc and soleus, which reach over to the medial side of the shin, and several strips of long, thin muscle with longer names than you need to worry about on the lateral side. The top of all the muscles on both sides of the shin attach to the knee. On the bottom, they attach to the tibia bone and foot.

As with the back of the leg, apply pressure as you slide toward the heart, and release on the way back to assist circulation.

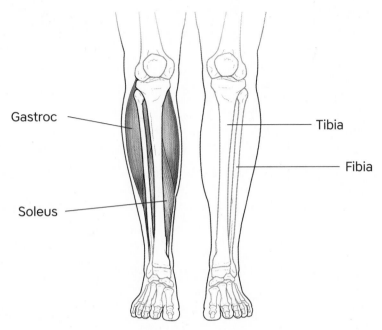

FIGURE 21: FRONT LOWER LEG

On Yourself

While sitting, place your fingers on the lateral side of the shin just below the knee. Flex your foot up and down to feel the muscles move. Slide down the leg, an inch or so at a time, continuing to flex and relax your foot, feeling the muscles. Repeat on the medial side of the shin. You'll notice the muscles on the medial side are smaller and less impressive than those on the lateral side. With your knuckles, scrape the muscles on both sides of the shin. As with the back of the calf, you'll notice that the tissue nearing the foot is more sensitive.

On Your Buddy

Fold back the massage sheet to just above the knee, and tuck between the lower legs. Without oil, palpate the length of the shin on both sides. Hold in several spots with one or both Duckbills, and ask your Buddy to flex and point their foot to feel these muscles move.

Face the calf, and spread oil over the shin and calves. Warm the area up by grabbing the shin with your Duckbill (use the arm closest to the foot) just above the ankle, thumb to the lateral side and fingers to the medial. Slide your hand all the way up and back down on each side of the shin. You'll notice that your thumb is on a long strip of muscle that lies right alongside the shin, all the way up to the knee. Give a little extra pressure on that muscle. Lift your hand, return to the ankle, and repeat several times, always moving in one direction, ankle to knee. This improves circulation in the lower leg.

Maintaining the same Duckbill position, grasp the shin just above the ankle, and press your thumb and fingers in circles on each side of the shin. Next, push those circles all the way up the shin, as if making a long line of loops. When you reach the top, lift your hand, return to just above the ankle, and repeat, always moving from ankle to knee.

Place the heels of your hands on either side of the shin, just above the ankle. Press into the heels to slide your palms all the way up both sides of the shin to just below the knee. Fold your fingers underneath both sides of the gastroc toward the back of the calf, and pull your palms firmly all the way back, grasping the heel to gently stretch the Achilles tendon. Return the heels of your hands to where you started, and repeat several times. On the last heel pull, release and slide your hands over the foot and brush the toes.

Cover the lower leg with the massage sheet, and repeat on the other side.

Cheat Sheet
FRONT OF THE LOWER LEG

To help you remember the sequence for the lower leg while faceup, write these steps in your notebook and place it where you can see it as you practice: Duckbill slides; Duckbill circles; palm slides up both sides of shin, palm pulls underneath gastroc, Achilles tendon stretch; slide over feet, brush toes.

Thigh

Like the back of the thighs, the front also offers a long, wide surface to work on. The muscles of the front of the thigh are often just called the "quads" collectively. Although the thigh looks like one big, impressive muscle on the outside, the quads are actually four muscles working together. For our purposes, we're treating them the way they look—like one big muscle. Underneath all that muscle in the middle of the leg is one long, strong bone called the femur, joining to the knee and hip at either end.

There is one muscle I want to highlight: the "sartorius," which is the long, thin muscle extending from the inner thigh to the outer hip. It's the longest muscle in the body, attaching to the top of the medial side of the tibia and the lateral side of the lower ilium. It rotates the thigh and lifts the leg up sideways. It's not so much what this muscle does as the angle of it that's important. You'll be following that angle for some of the thigh techniques. You can roughly remember it as running diagonally across the thigh from the medial side of the knee to the lateral side of the hip.

The "iliotibial tract," commonly known as the "IT band," is another one to note. It is a long band of fibrous tissue running from the lateral side of the knee to the lateral side of the hip, and oh, this can be one tight, painful little sucker, particularly for runners and cyclists, and it's often painful when we first start working it because it's so tight. When it's severely irritated, it can cause pain in the tendon (tendonitis) on the lateral side of the knee. This is another area where you must start with a light touch and add pressure very slowly and carefully.

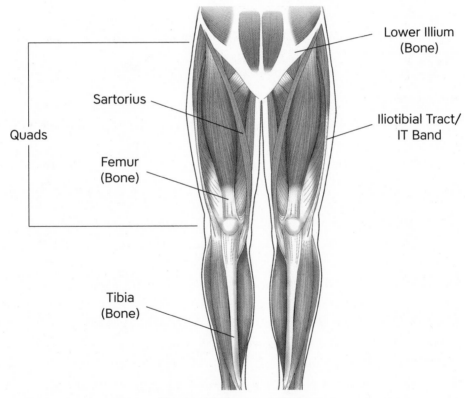

FIGURE 22: FRONT OF THIGH

On Yourself

While seated, lift and straighten your leg out in front of you, and place your palm on top of your thigh. Note how large and strong it is. Flex your foot up and down, and notice the thigh muscles don't move like the calf muscles did. That's because the main job of this group of muscles is to provide power and stability to the leg, and to stabilize the kneecap.

Put your foot back on the floor, and place the heel of your hand at the top center of the thigh, and lean on it to press down to just above the knee. Repeat with more pressure, noting that the quads can take a lot.

Run your Scraper up and down just above the knee to feel the thigh attachments. Scrub your knuckles back and forth, very firmly, from your greater trochanter to the lateral side of the knee. That itchy, burning sensation is your IT band.

Place your palm against the middle of your medial (inner) thigh, and press your thigh into your hand to feel your sartorius working. Drag and press your palm from outward to just below the greater trochanter to trace the angle of the sartorius.

Stand and put a palm on top of each thigh, and do some squats to feel the quads lifting and lowering your body. You'll also feel your glutes participating. These muscles all together are your powerhouse.

On Your Buddy

Roll the massage sheet back to expose the entire front of the leg. Tuck the sheet between the thighs, being extra careful not to expose or touch the genitals.

Without oil, palpate the surface of the thigh. Ask your Buddy to flex and release their quads so you can feel the muscles working. With both palms on top of the thigh, ask your Buddy to relax their thigh completely. Lean onto the heels of your hands slightly to rock and roll the muscle back and forth, and feel it slide over the femur. Jiggle it under your palms, continuing to note the movement of the muscle over the bone and the movement in the hip joint.

Place a palm firmly on the medial thigh, and ask your Buddy to press their thigh into your palm to locate the sartorius. Trace its angle to the upper lateral thigh. At the lateral side of the knee, scrub your knuckles up and down towards the hip, and ask your Buddy to let you know when they feel the itchy burn of the IT band.

Spread oil over the thigh, and do some palm slides to warm up. Open your Duckbills very wide to grasp the top of the thigh, a few inches apart, and slowly and deeply knead that big muscle with both hands. Swipe your palms in big, deep figure-eight circles over the quads, one after the other. Make nice big circles, like you're wiping a wet car.

With the hand closest to the foot, place your palm at the lower end of the sartorius on the medial side of the thigh. Press your palm over the quads along the angle of the sartorius to its upper attachment on the lateral side of the tibia. Let your hand slide off the side, lift your hand, return to start, and repeat. Try the same motion with your Steamroller, placing your elbow just above the lower end of the sartorius, your forearm angle toward the lateral side of the thigh, your fingers draping over, just as you did on the back of the thigh. Press your forearm only (not the elbow) over the quads to the upper end of the sartorius and slide off laterally just as you did with your palm. Lift, return to start, and repeat. Concentrate on keeping your glide slow. Experiment with the pressure for both the palm slide and Steamroller, and check in with your Buddy.

Place both Irons side by side on the IT band near the knee. Using them together like one big Iron, press lightly into the IT band and slide slowly to the top; release the pressure, and slide your Irons gently back to start. Repeat. Add pressure to this move in small increments, checking in with your Buddy about the pressure.

Finish by doing a couple more palm slides over the quads, and at the top of the last slide, slide down the length of the leg and over the top of the foot. Slide both palms at once all the way back up on both the medial and lateral side of the leg, and then back down the leg a couple times. On the last pass, brush your fingers over the toes.

Cover the leg with the sheet and repeat on the other side.

Cheat Sheet
THIGH (FRONT)

To help you remember the sequence for the front of the thigh, write these steps in your notebook and place it where you can see it as you practice: palm slide warmup; Duckbill kneading; "wipe the car" in figure eights; palm slides over quads; Steamroll quads; Iron IT band; palm slides over quads; palm slides over length of leg; brush toes.

All Together Now:
Foot, Lower Leg, Thigh

Just as we did with the back of the legs, practice the foot, lower leg, and thigh as one long combined sequence for the front of the leg: first one leg, then the other. The cheat sheet for the entire front of the leg is all the cheat sheets from each area, combined.

Stomach

People seem to either love or hate having their stomach massaged. Some find it very soothing, while others find it too intimate or embarrassing. I always ask a new person if it's okay to massage the stomach. If they say no, then it's no. I just skip this step and move on. This sequence (and actually, any sequence) can be omitted if your loved one doesn't want it.

Stomach massage is slow, gentle, and smooth. It's mostly to soothe, rather than to soften muscles. Lots of organs are nestled inside the abdominal cavity, so be extra careful and gentle when massaging there. Stomach moves are done in a clockwise direction, because the large intestine empties in a clockwise direction, and gentle clockwise palm circles may relieve constipation. Stomach massage can also ease menstrual cramps, and pregnant women often appreciate gentle work on the stomach. This is safe, with their physician's blessing; however, after the first trimester, a pregnant woman should lie on their side rather than their back.

When working on a female, draping the breast area before working on the stomach is mandatory. Place a folded pillowcase over the breast area, on top of the massage sheet. Anchor the pillowcase with one hand, and slowly tug the massage sheet free from underneath with the other. Fold the sheet back to the "bikini line." This is as low as you can go on anyone, male or female, while massaging the stomach.

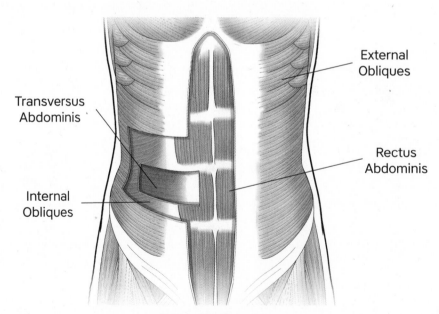

External Obliques

Transversus Abdominis

Rectus Abdominis

Internal Obliques

FIGURE 23: STOMACH

On Yourself

Lie on your back and palpate the bowl formed by the rib cage, and pubic and pelvic bones, with your belly filling that bowl. Run your palms in a clockwise circle slowly around your belly button. Tighten your abdominals and palpate to feel the muscles.

On Your Buddy

Stand facing the waistline. Spread some oil over the stomach, place your relaxed palms in the center of the stomach, and just hold. Breathe, and channel relaxation and comfort. Slide your palms simultaneously across the belly in opposite directions to each side of the waistline, back and forth, over and over, slowly, slowly.

Reach across the body with both hands, and place your palms on the waistline across from you. Curve your fingers a bit, and drag one hand after the other to the center line of the stomach, over and over, slowly, slowly. Place a palm in the center of the stomach, and circle around the table to the other side of the body. Repeat the back and forth slides, and the waistline pulls.

Place your palms on either side of the belly button, as if on a steering wheel. Make slow, gentle clockwise circles around the belly button, one hand following the other. Continue making palm circles until it feels comfortable and natural.

Place one palm above the belly button, one below, and slide them apart over the stomach, one toward the rib cage, the other toward the bikini line, giving the abdominal muscles a gentle stretch. Lift your hands, return to center, and repeat. Move the position of your palms just a bit each time you return so you cover the whole surface of the stomach, gently stretching and smoothing.

Place the massage sheet over the pillowcase covering the breasts, and gently tug the pillowcase free.

Cheat Sheet
STOMACH

To help you remember the sequence for the stomach, write these steps in your notebook and place it where you can see it as you practice: spread oil, place palms, hold, breathe; back-and-forth palm slides; waistline pulls; palm circles around belly button; slide palms apart and stretch.

Hands

Like the feet, the hands have lots of bones—twenty-seven in all; one more than the feet. There are thirty muscles in the hand, and over one hundred ligaments and tendons. Ligaments connect bone to bone, and tendons connect muscles to bone. Also like the feet, the hands get lots of daily wear and tear.

Although the hands and feet are shaped quite differently, the structures are similar. There's a cluster of chunky-shaped bones, as well as long bones and several joints. The chunkies below the wrist are the carpals. The long bones between the carpals and first row of knuckles are "metacarpals." The long bones of the fingers between each knuckle are "phalanges."

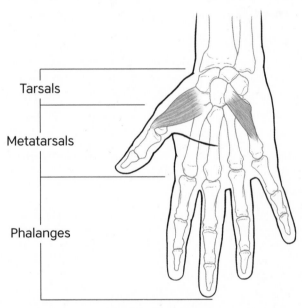

Tarsals

Metatarsals

Phalanges

FIGURE 24: HAND

On Yourself

We explored our hands in great detail already in chapter 7, so just revisit your magical hands briefly, and palpate to find the bones, joints, and soft tissue on the top of the hand and palm, as well as the thumb and each finger.

On Your Buddy

Without oil, explore and palpate the top of the hand and fingers, feeling for the bones, joints, and soft tissue. Spread oil over both sides of the hand. Hold the hand palm-down in one of your hands, and with the thumb and forefinger of your other hand, squeeze and slide between each metacarpal. Grasp the knuckle at the base of the index finger, and squeeze and squish your way to the fingertip. Give the little muscles between the knuckles some squishy-squeezies. Repeat on each finger and the thumb.

Pinch the web of the hand between your thumb and index finger. Pinch around the web to locate that sore, tight lump that most people have, then pinch and hold. Check in with your Buddy about the pressure. Pressing this spot can make your eyes water, but it really relieves tension in the hand and sometimes relieves headaches.

Turn the hand palm-up, and hold it in your laced fingers, your thumbs on the palm. With your thumbs, press and slide circles all over the palm.

Repeat on the other hand.

Cheat Sheet
HAND

To help you remember the sequence for the hand, write these steps in your notebook and place it where you can see it as you practice: squeeze and slide between metacarpals; squeeze and squish length of each finger and thumb; squeeze and squish little finger muscles; pinch web, press, and hold; thumb circles on palm.

Your arm has two sections: the lower arm or forearm, which has two bones (ulna and radius), and your upper arm, which has one (humerus). They join at the elbow. We use our arms constantly, often repetitively, and the muscles, tendons, and ligaments can get really tight and sore. Just as we aided circulation in the legs, so shall we do with the arms: when doing long slides and sweeping moves, apply pressure as you move toward the heart, and release as you move away from it.

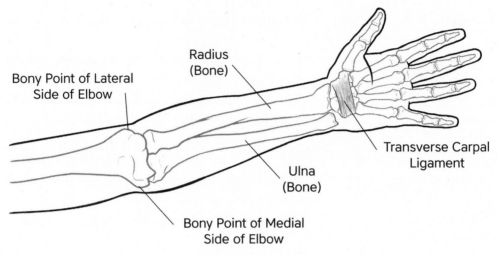

FIGURE 25: LOWER ARM

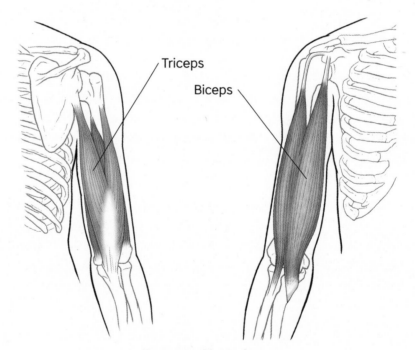

FIGURE 26: UPPER ARM

On Yourself

First, the forearm. Palpate to locate the two bones, and palpate the soft tissue over and between them. Support one arm on a table or place your hand on your knee. With the other, grab your wrist in your Duckbill, thumb underneath, just behind the heel of the hand. "Bite" hard with your Duckbill to feel the wide, flat ligament there. This is the "transverse carpal ligament," which can compress the medial nerve running underneath it, causing "carpal tunnel syndrome," which is very painful and interferes with the mobility and strength of the hand. It is caused by small, repetitive hand movement over time, such as typing, or working as a grocery cashier or dental hygienist.

Make Duckbill "bites" at one-inch intervals from the wrist to the elbow, pausing to really squeeze each one. Notice how these deep squeezes really relieve tension in your forearm.

Locate the bony bumps on the medial and lateral side of the elbow. Press your fingers in and roll circles all around these bumps. These bony points are actually the lower ends of each side of the humerus, where the tendons of the lower arm attach. Chronic pain and inflammation at these attachments is called "tendonitis." On the lateral side, it is "tennis elbow." On the medial side, it's "golfer's elbow." And you don't need to ever have held a tennis racket or golf club in your life to develop either. Again, it's all about repetitive motion over time. If these tendons feel tight and painful, grasp your upper forearm and rub your thumb deeply back and forth up and down the tendons. It often seems that the more painful the tendon, the more pressure they appreciate.

Now, the upper arm.

You know where your biceps is—that's the muscle that bulges up when you flex your arm. On the underside is the triceps, which can start to sag like a floppy fish belly as we age. To explore your upper arm, cross your arm over your chest and grab your bicep. Squeeze up and down and all around. Find the dip at the top of the biceps. Above this dip is the deltoid, which caps the point of the shoulder. Grab the deltoid and lift your arm, then rotate your arm in circles to feel it working.

On Your Buddy

There are two ways to work on the arm. One is to leave the arm lying flat on the table the whole time. The other is to lift and support the forearm while simultaneously working on it. The upper arm is gripped between your upper arm and rib cage to massage it.

To support the forearm, turn it palm-side up and grasp it at the wrist in both hands, thumbs on top. You can also turn it palm-side down, thumbs still on top. To massage the forearm, one hand holds the wrist while the other Duckbill slides up and back along the forearm. You can repeat the slides with one hand and hold with the other, or alternate them back and forth: slide and hold, change hands, slide and hold, etc.

To support the upper arm, face the table, and with your arm closest to the feet, pick up the wrist and place it between your other upper arm and rib cage. Squeeze your upper arm firmly against your rib cage to pin the wrist there, leaving both hands free to massage the upper arm. Ask your Buddy to relax their arm like a rag doll, completely limp, allowing you to provide all the support. People often try to "help" when you lift their arms. To prompt your Buddy to relax their arm, jiggle it gently and remind them, "Relax your arm." Move around a bit, and notice how firmly you can pin the arm and still have a lot of freedom to move. It should feel very tight and secure.

Practice just the lifting and supporting before beginning the arm sequences. If it's too difficult, you can do all the moves with the arm lying on the table. I will explain the sequences as if supporting the arm, but either way, the process is essentially the same.

Without oil, explore the structures of your Buddy's forearm, leaving it lying on the table for now. Find the bones, and palpate the soft tissue between them. Palpate for the tendons and attachments at the wrist and at the bony points of the elbow. "Bite" your Buddy's wrist in your Duckbill, and make firm, deep bites all the way up the forearm and back.

Spread oil over the forearm on all sides, and grasp it in both hands at the wrist, palm down, your thumbs on top. Grasp the wrist firmly in one hand, and with the other, thumb on top, squeeze a Duckbill up the length of the top of the forearm to the elbow, and back to the wrist. Repeat several times to warm and soften the tissue. Switch hands, and repeat using your opposite hands. Practice alternating your hands after each slide. Turn the forearm over, palm up, and repeat the whole process.

Place the forearm on the table, palm down, and press the heel of your hand just above the wrist and up the length of the forearm to the lateral point of the elbow, sliding off the lateral side. Lift your hand and return to start to slide again, always in one direction, from wrist to elbow.

Finish by swiping your relaxed palms up the forearm and back to the wrist. Repeat a couple times, and on the last pass, sweep down over the wrist, and grasp the hand, giving it a gentle pull to stretch the arm.

Moving to the upper arm, spread oil over the upper arm *before* pinning it to your side. Pin the wrist firmly between your upper arm and rib cage, and grasp the upper arm with both hands: big Duckbills to surround the whole upper arm on each side. Squeeze your

Duckbills up and down the length of the upper arm, one after the other, back and forth, like pistons. Spend some time here, warming and softening the biceps and triceps.

Place the arm on the table, and grasp the upper arm in both Duckbills, kneading across the muscle, from elbow to shoulder and back. With the heel of your palm, press all across the deltoid, from the bottom of the muscle to the point of the shoulder. Grab the whole deltoid in one hand and knead it like a big ball of dough.

Finish by sliding oil from the shoulder to the hand, then slide your palm back up from wrist to shoulder and back down again a couple times. On the last pass, slide down over the hand, and grasp it to pull gently, stretching the entire arm, just as you did when finishing the forearm.

Repeat the entire process on the other side.

Cheat Sheet
ARM

To help you remember the sequence for the hand, write these steps in your notebook and place it where you can see it as you practice: Duckbill bites on forearm; Duckbill forearm slides with one hand and then the other; Duckbill forearm slides with alternating hands; heel slides length of forearm; palm slides; gently pull hand; spread oil on upper arm; pin upper arm; big Duckbill slides; Duckbill kneading; deltoid presses; knead deltoid; palm slides along entire arm; gently pull hand.

All Together Now: Hands and Arms

Although we practiced on the hands and then the arms, in an actual massage, you'd move from the hand directly to the arm, then switch sides to repeat, starting over on the other hand and moving on to that arm. Practice going from the hand to the arm on each side. The cheat sheet is the cheat sheets for the hand and arm, combined.

Pectorals

Anyone who's ever seen a beefy man strut around without a shirt has seen nice bulging pectoral muscles. Well, women have pecs too, but much of that area is covered by our breasts. We'll be focusing on the area above the breasts and below the collarbones, for both men and women. On men, you can go a bit lower and deeper into the pectorals, but stay well above the nipple area. Nipples are no-no's.

The pectoral muscles span the upper chest, from under the collarbone at the shoulder to the medial humerus, and from the sternum (breastbone) and upper ribs to under the armpits. The pectoralis major is the large, thick upper layer that's easily visible, and underneath is the pectoralis minor. The pectorals control the movement of the arm and provide power for lifting weight, squeezing the arms together over the chest, and doing pushups.

Those with very physical jobs, like construction or masonry, or who spend a lot of time at the gym, can get tight, sore pecs, and may be surprised when you start working that area at how tender those big, strong muscles actually are. Even if you don't do lots of heavy, physical work, you may also be surprised!

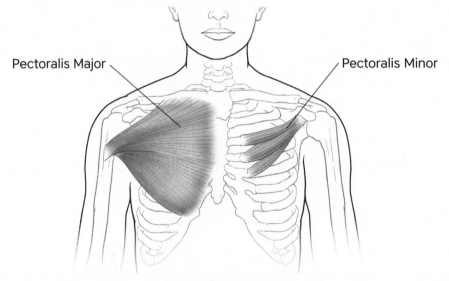

Pectoralis Major

Pectoralis Minor

FIGURE 27: PECTORALS

On Yourself

Cross one arm over your chest and grasp that big strip of muscle under the armpit. Move the arm up and down, rotate it, and push and pull to feel the muscles moving. Slide your Scraper from under your armpit to the collarbone, following the curve of the upper chest to the sternum. This is our work area for the pectorals.

On Your Buddy

At the end of the table, sit on a chair facing the head. Place both your palms on the pecs, one on each side of the sternum. Ask your Buddy to lift their forearms together over their chest to feel the muscles move.

Spread oil over both sides of the pecs simultaneously with your palms, each hand mirroring the other. Bring your palms together near the sternum, and push them outwards to the armpit, pressing into the heels. Swoop them back together and repeat, warming and softening. Repeat with your Irons.

Grab that strip of muscle below the armpit at the lateral sides of the chest, and knead it in your hands. Squish, squeeze, and soften.

Finish by spreading your palms from the sternum out over the upper pecs, following the curve under the collarbone. Continue swooping outward over the deltoid and slide both hands underneath the upper back, then pull them up to the tops of the shoulders. Each hand finishes in a Duckbill on top of the shoulders, thumbs on the front of the shoulder, fingers flat underneath the upper back. From here, we will move directly to the shoulders.

Shoulders

The top of the shoulder is actually the trapezius, coming up the back, and curling over the top to connect to the collarbone and also swooping up the back of the neck, attaching to the back of the skull. Hunch your shoulders up as tight as you can and tighten the back of the neck to feel the upper trapezius contracting. Underneath the trapezius at the top of the shoulder and back of the neck are other strips of muscle that lift and hunch the shoulders, and assist the pectorals when doing a pull-up and carrying heavy loads.

We learned about the shoulders and did the bulk of the work on them with your Buddy facedown, but there's a bit more we can do faceup. Accessing the upper shoulders and scapula area is sometimes easier with your Buddy faceup, because you can slide your hands underneath and dig your fingers into the muscle while sliding up, using the person's body weight to apply pressure. A flat hand sliding down and up under the body is also very effective. However, while faceup, the bulk of the shoulder work is on the top, which is the upper end of the trapezius, running from the collarbone to the back of the skull.

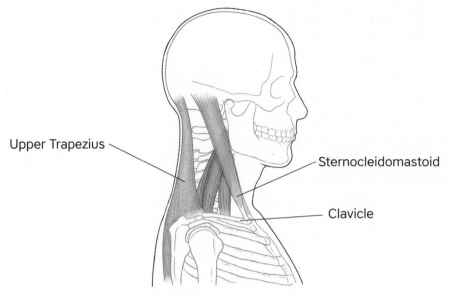

Upper Trapezius

Sternocleidomastoid

Clavicle

FIGURE 28: FRONT OF SHOULDER

On Yourself

You already explored the shoulder area on yourself in the last chapter, so we'll jump directly to practicing on your Buddy. You can repeat the shoulder exploration on yourself if you wish.

On Your Buddy

Seated behind your Buddy's head, pick up directly where you left off at the pectorals, one shoulder in each Duckbill, thumbs on top. The top of the shoulders is in your palms, your flat fingers underneath on the upper back. Squeeze the shoulders, and ask your Buddy to scrunch their shoulders up to their ears and release, to feel the contraction and release of the muscles. Grab the roll of muscle on each side, and jiggle it firmly to loosen the area.

Add more oil if necessary, and knead both sides deeply and slowly in your Duckbills, alternating one hand after the other, over and over. Really dig in and add some pressure, and dig into the upper back with your fingers too. This is one of those moves that makes people swoon. Take your time, and get the shoulders nice and warm and soft.

Put the heels of your hands at the base of the neck on each side, fingers pointing toward the tips of the shoulders, and deeply press the heel to slide it along the top of the shoulder from the neck to where the collarbone joins the shoulder. While returning that hand to start, press the heel of the other hand out over the top of the other shoulder. One hand slides as the other returns. Slide and return, slide and return, over and over. Repeat this move with your Irons. Ask your Buddy about the pressure, and experiment with how much the shoulders can actually take, and enjoy.

Press your Irons straight into the top of the shoulders, and alternately push deeply into them, back and forth, as if they're slowly marching in place.

Return to the double Duckbill shoulder kneading you started with, even deeper this time, one hand after the other.

To finish the shoulders, slide your palms as far down underneath the upper back as is comfortable for you. Curl and press your fingers into the back, letting the weight of the body provide the pressure. If your Buddy lifts their chest to "help," gently remind them to relax into your hands. Drag your fingers and palms, both hands at once, up the upper back, over the top of the shoulders, and then swoop both palms away from each other, out over the point of each shoulder.

Finish this combined sequence by revisiting the pectorals: Swoop both palms over the pecs, then out over the deltoids, up over the points of the shoulders, and then slide your palms along the tops of the shoulders and on up the sides of the neck, stopping with the head cradled in your hands. From here, you will transition directly to the neck.

Cheat Sheet
PECTORALS AND SHOULDERS

To help you remember the sequence for the pectorals and shoulders while faceup, write these steps in your notebook and place it where you can see it as you practice: palm slides across pectorals; Iron pectorals; squeeze pectorals below armpits; palm slides out over pectorals and deltoids, and up shoulder tops, ending in Duckbill on shoulders; Duckbill kneads on shoulders; heel slides along shoulder tops; Iron shoulder tops; Iron "marching" on shoulder tops; deep Duckbill kneads; palm slides from underneath back to shoulders, and outward along shoulder tops; palm slides over pectorals and deltoids, over top of shoulder and up sides of neck, stopping at head.

Neck

The neck seems to give everyone misery. The more time spent hunched over a keyboard or with chronic poor posture, the more this is so. Hunching your back and collapsing your chest really puts stress on your neck. The "fast pass" to relieving neck pain is to improve posture: roll your shoulder blades up and over, slide them down your back, and imagine your chest and head are being lifted up by strings, rather than leaving the back to do all the work of supporting the torso. When you leave it up to your back to support your torso, it often slouches into a hunch.

Before working on anyone's neck, ask if they've had a neck injury, surgery, or condition that require you to be extra gentle, particularly when lifting or turning the head. Before practicing on the neck, study the graphic carefully to find the sternocleidomastoid muscle. This is one muscle we must know, and be able to identify. Forget the fancy name, just remember its initials, S.M., which also means "Stop Muscle." The Stop Muscles runs from the medial tip of the collarbone to base of the skull behind the ear. You can work on it, or behind it—never in front of it. All soft tissue in front of the Stop Muscle toward the throat, and the throat itself, are off limits.

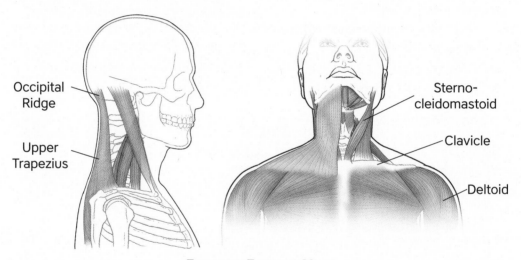

FIGURE 29: FRONT OF NECK

On Yourself

Turn your head over one shoulder as far as you can, and trace the length of your Stop Muscle. It will feel like a tight rope stretching from your clavicle to the bottom of your skull, just behind your ear. Notice how this muscle forms a triangle with the clavicle and the top of your shoulder. This is your working zone for the neck, within that triangle *only*. If you gently probe over the Stop Muscle toward the throat, you'll immediately see how uncomfortable this is. Stay inside the triangle.

We already explored the neck in the last chapter, so we'll jump straight to practicing on your Buddy. You can revisit the self-exploration of the neck before continuing if you wish.

On Your Buddy

Begin the faceup sequence for the neck right where you left off at the sequence for the pectorals and shoulders, with your hands cradling the head. Your fingers will be near the occipital ridge, which forms the bottom edge of the back of the skull, and feels like a little speed bump. Run your fingertips firmly up and down over that little speed bump. Slide the fingers of both hands down each side of the neck, and slide back to the head. Repeat a few times. Rub gentle circles over both sides of the neck with your fingertips, feeling the tight muscles there.

Gently slide one palm back under the head, holding it in your palm. Cross your other hand over the face, and gently place your palm on the side of the forehead. Turn the head by slowly pressing against the forehead while simultaneously curling the fingers underneath to pull the head. Turn the head only to the first point of resistance—no further. Some people can turn their heads almost over their shoulders, and others only a little bit. Never force the neck to turn. Work within its limitations.

Now, you will switch hands under the head, and cradle it in the other palm. Your other hand is now free to work on the side the head is turned away from. With your free hand, rub your fingers along the borders of your safe working triangle, formed by the top of the shoulder, clavicle, and Stop Muscle. Apply some oil, and slide your fingers in soft, flat circles all over this triangle, warming it up.

Slide your fingers along the top of the shoulder and up the back of the neck to locate the trapezius. Experiment with your Scraper, Iron, and knuckles to warm up this muscle. As you massage this area, recall the graphic of the neck, and imagine the muscles, tendons, and bones under your hands. Work on the soft tissue next to the cervical spine *only*, not on the cervical spine itself.

Grasp the whole neck in your free hand, thumb on one side of the neck, fingers on the other, and knead those tight muscles on the side of the neck, over and over, as if smooshing hard clay slowly and deeply in your hand. Stay there for a bit, then smoosh all the way down the top of the shoulder, and smoosh a bit more between the clavicle and shoulder.

Make a soft fist, and slide your relaxed knuckles up and down on the side of the neck a few times, then slide your knuckles down the side of the neck and out over the top of the shoulder. Slide them back up to just below the head, and then back out over the top of the shoulder again. Repeat several times.

Place the heel of your free hand at the side of the neck, just under the ear. Holding the head firm with the other hand underneath, press the heel of your hand down the side of the neck and over the top of the shoulder, stopping just before where the clavicle joins it. Lift your hand, and return to start. Repeat this move in long, slow slides, always in one direction—head to shoulder. Experiment with increasing the pressure of your slide. The muscle on top of the shoulder appreciates deeper pressure. Repeat the same one-way slide with your Iron. Also, experiment with tilting the head away from the shoulder a bit with the hand supporting it. This creates a longer plane over the top of the shoulder, giving it a nice stretch.

Slide your free hand under the head, palm up, and cradle the head. Slide the other hand out, and repeat the entire sequence on the other side.

Finish the neck by repeating the same sequence for finishing the pectorals and shoulders: Swoop both palms over the pecs, out over the deltoids and over the points of the shoulders, then along the tops of the shoulders and on up the sides of the neck to cradle the head in both palms. From here, you transition directly to the scalp. For all remaining sequences from this point forward, it's no longer necessary to use oil unless your Buddy prefers it.

Cheat Sheet
NECK
———

To help you remember the sequence for the neck while faceup, write these steps in your notebook and place it where you can see it as you practice: massage occipital ridge; fingertip circles on both sides of neck; turn head and apply oil; circles over triangle; fingers, Scraper, Iron, and knuckles along top of shoulder and back of neck; knead and smoosh neck; knead and smoosh top of shoulder; soft knuckle slides on side of neck, then include top of shoulder; heel slides from side of neck down over top of shoulder; Iron from side of neck down over top of shoulder; switch hands; finish by swooping over pecs, deltoids, shoulders, and up neck, stopping to cradle head in palms.

Scalp

A scalp massage feels luscious, particularly for those with long, thick, heavy hair. All that hair pulls on the scalp! Even without any hair at all, a scalp massage feels great because the scalp is much more than skin covering the cranium. The skin has more than what's on the surface: thin layers of muscle, connective tissue, blood vessels, and fat.

On Yourself

Lie down on your back, lace your hands behind your head, and slide your thumbs up to the bottom edge of your skull to find that little speed bump—the occipital ridge. The scalp muscles anchor here, as does the upper trapezius of the neck. When your trapezius muscles are chronically tense, it makes the soft tissue over the occipital ridge tight and sore. Slide your thumbs firmly up and down over your occipital ridge. Holy cow, right? You probably didn't even realize you were sore there. Your loved one probably doesn't either. Press your thumbs in slow, deep circles over your occipital ridge to experience the relief this provides.

Tighten and release your hands, which will pull your fingertips back and forth across your scalp on the back of your head, and your thumbs up and down over the occipital ridge. As you tighten and release movement, slide your hands to the top of your head. Continue tightening and releasing, and deepen the pressure with your thumbs and fingers to experience how wonderful this deep, back-and-forth massage feels on the scalp. You can even experience that "delicious ache" on the scalp.

Lighten the pressure until your fingers and thumbs scrub very gently over the skin and hair. Now, holding your hands stationary, press very deeply into the scalp, until you can slide it over your skull. It will only slide a little bit. Discover its range of motion by sliding your scalp back and forth over your skull, sideways, in circles and in figure eights. Finish by giving your scalp a gentle scratchy scrub all over with your fingernails, and enjoy that tingly feeling.

On Your Buddy

Picking up from where you left off at the neck, the head cradled in your palms, notice that your hands are in a different position than when you practiced on yourself: now, the fingertips are on the occipital ridge, and your thumbs are on the sides of the head.

Press and slide your fingers in unison all along the occipital ridge. Rotate your hands underneath the head to lace the fingers behind the head, then slide the fingers back and forth sideways across the back of the head like pistons. Massage the scalp all over with your fingertips. Experiment with the pressure.

Slide your thumbs to the top of the head, then back and forth next to each other all over the top of the head. Press your palms into the top of the head, fingers draping down the sides, and slide the scalp over the skull, back and forth, in circles, and in figure eights.

Finish with light, luxurious nail scratching all over the scalp, and then drag your fingertips through the hair to the ends.

Ears

We may just think of our ears as convenient places to hang our hoops, but the outer ears have much more to offer: massaging them until they're soft and warm feels heavenly. Ears are also great because you can massage the ears on most anyone, regardless of position or clothing. All jewelry and plugs must be removed before working on the ears.

On Yourself

Squeeze the earlobe between the sides of your curled index fingers and your thumbs, your thumbs on the back side. Squeeze circles all over the lobe, then pull down on the lobes slowly and firmly. Flip your hands over so your thumbs are now on the fronts of your ears, and squeeze circles all over the outer curls of the ear until they feel warm and squishy. Grasp your outer ears between your thumbs and index fingers, and pull outwards, away from your head.

On Your Buddy

As you grasp your Buddy's ears between your thumbs and curled index fingers, notice that your thumbs and fingers are opposite of how you explored your own ears because your hands are in a different position now. Your thumbs will be on top of the earlobes, fingers underneath, and you won't have to flip them over to massage the outer ear curls. Your hands will work in unison.

Repeat all the movements you did on your own ears. Finish by giving the earlobes a long, loving, smooshy squeeze between your thumbs and fingers.

Cheat Sheet
SCALP AND EARS

To help you remember the sequence for the scalp and ears, write these steps in your notebook and place it where you can see it as you practice: finger slides over occipital ridge; slide fingers back and forth under head; all-over fingertip massage; thumb slides on top of head; press scalp over skull; scratch; drag through hair; squeeze circles on earlobes; pull lobes; circle squeezes on outer ear curls; pull ears away from head; smooshy squeeze.

Jaw

The main muscle of the jaw, called the masseter, is the most powerful in the body, allowing us to bite and chew. An adult human bite can exert 110 to 150 pounds of force, and is capable of exerting a maximum of 275 pounds of force. That seems like a lot, but a lion can exert 1,234 pounds of force in its bite! And that's nothing compared to a full-grown saltwater crocodile, which can bite with 3,700 pounds of pressure!

Luckily, we don't have to catch and kill prey with our jaws. We mostly just do a lot of chewing. The masseter can get sore over time, as can the joint of the jaw, which can even develop arthritis. A common affliction of the jaw is "temporomandibular joint dysfunction" (and isn't that, ironically, a mouthful!), which most of us call "TMJ." Massaging the masseter can provide some relief for TMJ.

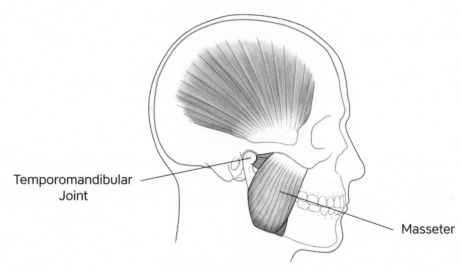

Temporomandibular Joint

Masseter

FIGURE 30: JAW AND SCALP

On Yourself

Place your fingertips on your jaw just below your cheekbones, and clench your teeth to feel the masseter bulge out. Open and close your mouth, then move your jaw from side to side, to feel this muscle working. Press your Scrapers into that bulge, and circle in one direction all over your masseters, then go in the other direction. Scrape down from the center of the masseter to the back corner of your jawbone, pulling the tissue down slowly and firmly under your braced fingertips.

For many people (including myself), pressing into the masseter and tissue below it, just behind the jawbone where the ear attaches to the neck, will trigger a gagging or coughing reflex. Press your fingers around that spot to see if you are also a gagger.

On Your Buddy

Place your fingers on both sides of your Buddy's face in unison, about where you imagine their back molars meet on each side of their jaw. Ask them to clench their jaw to find their masseter. Press your Scrapers into the masseter firmly, and do circles in both directions. Scrape from the masseter to the bottom of the jaw, careful to avoid the gaggy spot.

Finish by placing your palms along the jawbone on both sides of the face, fingertips meeting at the chin. Sweep your hands slowly and lovingly back over the jawbone. From here, you transition directly to the face.

Face

We become so obsessed with the surface of our faces, we forget that there's a lot going on under the skin as well—lots of little muscles that are also soothed by touch. Before moving to the face, wipe your hands on the massage sheet to remove any residual oil. You can move the skin on the face and slide it over the facial bones, but don't stretch the skin. The orbit bones around the eyes form the eye sockets, and are your boundaries for working near the eyes. Never massage within the eye socket, or press into the eyes.

The face is our last stop before finishing the sequence for the front of the body, and also for a full-body massage. The face is where we begin to rejoin our Sacred Massage ritual. Therefore, the face sequence is slow, gentle, calming, and soothing. Although most people find facial massage relaxing, others just don't like it. If your loved one isn't a fan, no big deal. Skip the facial sequence entirely, and swap the jaw and scalp sequences: do the jaw after the neck, then the scalp, and finish the physical portion of the massage cradling the head in your palms.

On Yourself

Place the pads of your fingertips in the center of each cheek. Holding the skin in place with your fingertips, gently slide the cheek tissue in slow circles over the bones underneath. Circle one way, and then the other.

Slide your fingertips down the jawbone to your chin, and slowly slide the chin in circles over the bone underneath, first one way, then the other.

Slide your fingertips up to your temples, and massage gently in circles, letting the fingertips slide over the skin, just in one direction.

Massage your forehead with your fingertips, sliding the skin over the bone up and down, back and forth, and in circles in both directions.

On Your Buddy

Place your fingertips lightly in the center of the cheeks, and slide the cheeks in gentle circles over the bone, both directions. Both hands will move in unison for the entire facial sequence. Slide fingertips down the jaw to the chin, and circle the chin over the bone, both directions. Slowly, lightly massage the forehead with your fingertips, up and down, back and forth, and in circles.

Slide your fingertips up to the temples, and make long, slow, luxurious circles over the skin with your fingertips. As you're doing these temple circles, concentrate on bringing the energy down, down, down, and imagine your Buddy relaxing even deeper. Breathe slowly, deeply, and effortlessly. Temple circles are the transition point for inviting your awareness of yourself back into the massage session, front and center. Let love, compassion, and healing flow from your heart through your hands. Align your own serenity with your Buddy's, as if you're one connected, peaceful, divine channel.

When you feel spiritually present and connected, slide your hands underneath the head, cradling it in your palms. Breathe slowly and deeply into and out of your belly button. Become aware of your feet firmly grounded on the earth, and continue cradling the head, letting it rest. Really connect to your own spirit, your Buddy's, and the divine, magical energy of the universe. That energy flows freely between you, your Buddy, and Spirit.

Cheat Sheet
JAW AND FACE

To help you remember the sequence for the jaw and face, write these steps in your notebook and place it where you can see it as you practice: press circles over masseter, first one way, then the other; scrape from masseter to bottom corner of jaw; slide palms along jawline; press light circles in center of cheeks; slide chin in circles; forehead massage; circle temples while reconnecting to your breath, body, and spirit; slide hands under head to cradle it; breathe, rest, and connect.

Let Them Drift

The gentle, soothing facial work at the end of a massage often puts people to sleep. That's okay. Let them snooze. Sometimes when people fall asleep during massage, it's not true sleep but a "neither here nor there" place we call "golden slumber." It feels like drifting along on a heavenly cloud, your mind randomly wandering, a bit like light dreaming. If you spoke to someone in golden slumber, they'd respond. However, sometimes people do fall sound asleep, even snoring, and that's okay too. Sleep is what they needed most at that moment. If your Buddy falls asleep during the facial massage—or at any other point during the massage—let them drift. Don't make any quick movements or sounds that might wake them up. Let them just tip over that edge, and rest.

Finishing, Reconnecting, Returning

Congratulations! You know enough basic massage sequences to put them all together and do one smooth, flowing full-body sequence, which we'll practice in the next chapter. We'll also make the transition to a complete Sacred Massage ritual.

After finishing the face, your Buddy's head cradled in your palms, your focus on physical massage techniques and sequences transitions to the spiritual, magical, and divine: Sacred Massage. It's a bit like an airplane flight. We take off with a spiritual, magical focus, level out into physical Soothing Touch techniques for the flight, then land with a return to a spiritual, magical focus.

In the next chapter, you'll pull everything together in one smooth Sacred Massage experience, from beginning to end. Baby, you are ready for takeoff!

Chapter 10

Bringing It All Together in Sacred Massage

Can you believe it? You're ready to combine everything you've learned into a full-body routine! You may not *feel* ready, but you are. Feel the unreadiness, and do it anyway! First, we'll learn massage techniques for the entire body, and then we'll see how they fit into the overall Sacred Massage experience, from beginning to end: one cohesive, spiritual, magical, divine healing ritual. In this chapter, we'll blend the three parts of magic—intention, implementation, and manifestation—right into the structure of the massage routine. The massage itself becomes a magical ritual.

As before, we'll assume that you're working on a massage table, and that your Buddy is facedown for the back of the body, and faceup for the front. Your Buddy will be covered with a massage sheet, and has their ankles supported facedown, and their knees supported while faceup. The support is always under the bottom sheet, not touching the skin.

When you actually start massaging your loved one, they may not be in this position. That's okay. Learn the sequence in this position until it becomes familiar, and then adapt it later on for whatever position your loved one will be in. We'll go over some ways to customize your loved one's body position or physical circumstances at the end of this chapter.

Activity
RITUAL TO CLEANSE AND DEDICATE YOUR HEALING HANDS

Before we begin learning the Sacred Massage routine, let's first set a magical tone by doing a simple ritual to cleanse and dedicate the most precious, valuable magical tools of all: your hands. Let's really focus upon bringing all that magical, divine, healing energy online, and welcome it right into your hands and touch.

First, create a simple mantra just for your hands, such as "May compassion, comfort, and healing flow through my hands." Next, create an altar for honoring your hands and blessing them with skill, strength, compassion, divine healing, and magic. Your massage table would be perfect for this. Adorn your altar with items that represent those qualities to you—colors, crystals, or symbols.

For your ritual, you'll need a small bowl of salt, a large bowl of water, a table-spoon of magically significant crushed herb (fresh or dried) in a small bowl, olive oil, incense that represents healing energy, a white candle, matches, and a hand towel.

With everything in place, cast your magical circle clockwise around your altar with a stream of white light, and welcome the directions or elements, beginning at north, holding up your open palms. Welcome the God and Goddess with your palms, and represent them by placing your right index finger into the palm of your cupped left hand. Welcome your healing deity, with open palms, and bring your palms to your heart.

Place your palms on the altar and breathe. Ground and center.

Hold the candle and speak your mantra into it: "May compassion, comfort, and healing flow through my hands." Light it and set it on your altar. Light the incense, speak the same into it, and set it on your altar.

Rub some olive oil over your hands, and give them a nice massage. Put some salt into your palms, and rub the salt around and work it into the oil. Imagine the oil and salt purifying and protecting your hands as you gently massage all over them and through your fingers. This is mildly exfoliating, and you can imagine all negative energy sloughing away with any dry or dead skin cells. Rinse in the water, blot dry with the towel.

Drizzle a little olive oil into the crushed herb and stir clockwise with your finger until it's the consistency of paste. Chant some of the qualities of that herb as you stir. For example, if using rosemary, chant "protection, health, and healing." Luxuriously and lovingly massage the herb paste all over your hands, and imagine them soaking in that herb's energy. Channel love and appreciation to your marvelously talented hands. Invite your healing deity to bless those hands, and use them for channeling divine healing energy and compassion. Rinse in the water, blot dry with the towel.

Put your hands in prayer position, and draw them to your heart chakra. Close your eyes and say, "May the divine in me see the divine in everyone I touch." Tip your forehead toward your hands and say, "Namaste."

Wave your hands slowly through the incense smoke, and say, "So mote it be."

Rest in this special moment for as long as you like, letting yourself well up with a newfound appreciation for your healing hands. When you feel ready, thank your deity for participating and blessing your hands, thank the God and Goddess for their presence, and thank each of the directions, beginning at north, and moving counterclockwise. Uncast your circle by "vacuuming" the circle of white light back into your index finger, counterclockwise from north.

Your magical circle is now open, and your ritual is finished. You might never see your hands the same way again—the finest, most valuable magical tools you'll ever use.

With your healing hands energized, you're now ready to transfer that magic to your Buddy and learn the Sacred Massage routine.

Activity
'JUST SPREAD THE OIL' SEQUENCES

Your massage area prepared, and your Buddy situated on the table, our first practice will simply be to experience the flow and rhythm of a full-body massage routine. Forget about sequences, forget about tools and techniques, forget about bones and muscles and tendons. For our first practice, we won't worry about any techniques. Instead, we'll just be present in the experience of sliding your hands over another person's body. You'll cover the surface of the skin, and feel the shape of the body—all the curves and angles, the ridges and indentations.

Let your mind relax, and focus only on your hands and what they're feeling, at that moment in time. Clear your mind completely, and let your brain go all relaxed and dreamy. Imagine that your consciousness is in your hands. Let them softly, slowly slide and drag over the skin like warm, wet washcloths. Notice how warm they become. They feel heavy and completely relaxed. Imagine that you're not merely spreading oil over the skin—you're spreading pure liquid love, compassion, and relaxation.

After finishing the neck faceup, ditch the oil, and proceed with the remaining sequences by gently gliding your fingertips over each area.

Here we go.

Buddy Facedown

Stand facing the torso, and place your palms on the back. Clear your mind, breathe, and transfer your awareness into your hands. Fold sheet down to tailbone, slowly spread oil over back, then shoulders, then neck; unfold sheet and cover torso.

Lift sheet from one foot, tuck sheet between legs, and spread oil over sole. Continue with calf, then thigh. Spread oil over entire leg and sole. Cover leg with sheet. Rest palms on glutes, over sheet. Lift sheet from other foot, and repeat. Remove support from under feet.

Make "tent" with massage sheet, and direct your Buddy to turn over, and scoot down onto the table and out of the face cradle. Set face cradle aside. Realign body if necessary.

Buddy Faceup

Lift knees with one arm, and slide support under knees with the other. Smooth and straighten sheet; fold top edge down to collarbones if necessary.

Lift sheet from one foot, tuck between legs, and spread oil over foot. Continue with lower leg, and thigh. Spread oil over entire leg and foot. Cover leg with sheet. Lift sheet from other foot, and repeat. Cover leg with sheet.

Uncover arm, and spread oil over hand and fingers, then forearm, then upper arm. Cover with sheet. Uncover other arm, and repeat. Cover with sheet. Fold top edge of sheet down to armpits.

Sit in chair at end of massage table, behind head. Spread oil over pectorals. Spread oil over tops of shoulders. Spread oil over sides of neck. Wipe excess oil onto massage sheet.

Glide fingertips under head, up sides, and all over scalp. Slide fingertips gently through hair. Gently feel the earlobes and outer curls of the ears. Glide fingertips over masseter and jaw. Glide fingertips over cheeks, chin, forehead, and temples. Slide palms underneath head. Cradle head. Hold. Breathe.

Besides experiencing just "being" in your hands for this exercise, this extremely light Soothing Touch may be appropriate if your loved one is very delicate or frail, or has fibromyalgia or osteoporosis. It would also be appropriate for an infant. Gently slides all over the body, fueled by your love and compassion, could serve as your entire Soothing Touch sequence. Also, some people actually prefer a featherlight approach. If your loved one only wants to be soothed rather than have deeper massage work, just give them what they want. Remember, this is *their* massage session, not yours.

Adding On

Next, we'll add on to the "spread the oil" sequence we just did, bit by bit. Do these three practice sessions as described, repeating the entire sequence as before.

Review the graphics in the last two chapters before beginning. While repeating the "spread the oil" full-body sequence, visualize the muscles, bones, and tendons underneath the skin as your hands pass over these areas. Don't bother with names. Just remember the image of the bone or soft tissue, noticing how they feel under your palms. Imagine that you have x-ray vision and can see right through the skin as you proceed.

Repeat the entire "spread the oil" sequence, adding in the "Three P's" in each area as you go: Palpate (just feel around), Petrissage (knead the soft tissue like bread dough, one hand after the other, like a cat), and Press (use palms, fingers, and thumbs).

Review the "manual tools" and techniques in chapter 6. Go freestyle, and experiment with whichever ones you wish as you spread the oil. We only covered some basic ways to use tools and techniques, and there are many more ways to use them. Give any or all of the tools and techniques a whirl, and see which ones work well in which areas, and which don't. Don't worry about following the exact sequence for each area. Just play and explore. Find out which tools and techniques you prefer. When toying with your tools and techniques, ask your Buddy to provide feedback about how it feels.

Activity
FULL-BODY MASSAGE ROUTINE

Are you ready? Let's *do* this!

We'll work from an outline to practice the full-body routine, rather than reexplaining each sequence. Remember those cheat sheets you made for each area? If they aren't already in a spiral-bound notebook, place them in order in a binder or tack them to the wall to help you remember each sequence as you go along. If you forget something or get lost, no worries—just look at your cheat sheet.

Rather than worrying about memorizing sequences or techniques, just use your cheat sheets for as long as you like, even while working on your loved one if necessary. Eventually, the routines will sink into memory organically. The more you practice the full-body sequence, the sooner that will happen. One day, you'll realize you just did the whole routine without bothering to look at your notes. Think of your cheat sheets like training wheels—one day you just won't need them anymore, and you'll leave them behind and peddle away effortlessly.

Keep a pen or pencil handy to make notes on your cheat sheets. You may want to add or subtract, or change the order of the sequence. The ultimate goal isn't to copy my routine lockstep, and learn *my* dance. The goal is to take my full-body template and transform it into your own dance. When you've developed a routine you like, you might want to rewrite a fresh, new set of cheat sheets with the techniques you prefer.

To keep your book from turning into a wad of oily goo, copy the following full-body routine outline into your notebook, or write the outline on a large piece of paper or poster board and tack it to the wall so you can glance up at it to follow along. Keep your cheat sheets handy in case you need to jog your memory about a certain sequence.

Back

Make contact: palms on back, breathe.

Gentle warmup: brush body with fingertips, rock entire length of body with relaxed hands, rock torso on both sides with heels of hands next to spine.

Fold back massage sheet to tailbone. Spread oil on back, warm and soften tissue. Do back sequence on both sides. Do facedown sequence for shoulders and scapulae. Do facedown sequence for neck.

Cover back with sheet, and uncover the following as necessary. Do sequences for sole, calf, thigh, and glutes on one side, then the other. Cover legs with sheet. Remove support from under feet, set aside.

Lift sheet into a tent, ask Buddy to turn over onto their back, replace sheet. Help Buddy align themselves on the table if necessary. Lift legs at knees, slide support back under bottom massage sheet underneath knees.

Front

Smooth wrinkles from sheet, and check in: "How are you doing?" "Everything OK?"

Do sequence for top of foot, front of calf, and thigh on one side. Repeat on other side.

Prepare to do the stomach: cover breast area with pillowcase, pulling sheet down from underneath to bikini line. Do stomach sequence. Cover stomach and chest with sheet, remove pillowcase.

Do sequence for hand, forearm, and upper arm on one side. Repeat on other side. Do sequence for pectorals. Do faceup sequence for shoulders. Do faceup sequence for neck. Do scalp sequence. Do ear sequence. Do jaw sequence. Do face sequence. Cradle head in palms. Breathe.

Passing Time

A typical massage session lasts an hour. For a professional massage therapist, time matters because that's what your client expects, and is paying for. For a non-professional working on a loved one, time is less relevant. If your loved one only wants a 15-minute massage, that's fine. If they want you to go and go and go until you collapse, that's okay too, if it's okay with you.

You could do the entire full-body sequence at your own pace, and nobody but you or your loved one may care how long that takes. So, why are we talking about time at all? Because constraining your full-body practice sequence within an hour will teach you to pace yourself. If you breeze through a full-body sequence in thirty minutes, you're probably moving much too quickly. Conversely, if an hour has passed by and your Buddy hasn't turned over yet, you'll need to trim down your routine, rather than speeding up your pace.

Sometimes it helps to count the number of repetitions you do to keep your pace. I actually find that absent-minded counting as I go along keeps my mind free of unhelpful, distracting chatter. The slow counting becomes a meditation of sorts. Try doing each move seven times and count as you go if you're having trouble determining how fast or slow your pace is. You want to be at the slow end. A slow pace is more relaxing and soothing and allows you to safely press deeper or add pressure if necessary. Don't go buzzing along like you're waxing a car. Keep it *slooowwwww.*

Repeat the entire full-body sequence, using a clock to pace your speed. A clock is better than a timer because you can see the hands or numbers move as you go, rather than you and your Buddy being surprised by the timer going off.

Here is about how long you should spend on each area for a typical full-body massage:

Facedown: Warmup, back, shoulders, neck: fifteen minutes. Foot, leg, and glutes: five minutes on each side.

Faceup: Foot and leg, four minutes on each side. Belly, two minutes. Hand and arm, three minutes on each side. Pecs, shoulders, and neck, ten minutes. Scalp, ear, jaws, face, and finishing, eight minutes.

You might have noticed this comes to fifty-nine minutes. That's to allow a little wiggle room for your Buddy to turn over and get settled before proceeding to the front. You'll also notice that—holy cow!—when you break it down, it doesn't seem like much time for each area! It really is, though—it's all about practice. Once you feel confident that your pace is slow and controlled, unless there's a need to keep your massage session within a certain time frame, you don't need to pay any attention to the clock anymore.

How Did It Go?

Did you stay within the allotted time for each area? Did you stay within an hour for the full-body sequence? If yes, fantastic. If not, where did you head off into the weeds? Did you forget to do some of the moves? Did you go too fast or too slow? Were you able to find a slow, relaxed pace, or were you rushing to beat the clock? If a certain sequence gave you trouble, practice just that one again to evaluate whether you need to slow down or speed up that particular sequence to stay within the time constraint for that area.

If you did all the moves for each sequence and had a lot of time left, you must *slooooooow dooowwwwwn.* If you're certain you weren't moving too quickly, you can stretch any sequence by repeating moves, adding more tools, doing some petrissage, or just gliding and sliding with your palms.

Now, let's imagine the opposite situation.

If you found yourself running out of time for each sequence, or the whole full-body routine, rather than speeding up, do fewer repetitions of each move. Don't change your pace. Little bits trimmed from here and there add up to the amount of time you need to cut to stay on time. In a pinch, you could even drop a move for one or more sequences to stay within an hour.

Make Your Massage Sacred

Now that you've learned a basic full-body massage routine (which is also the "implementation" step for your magical massage ritual), we'll plug this into the comprehensive Sacred Massage experience, continuing with the magical ritual template.

The spiritual, magical tone of Sacred Massage begins as you prepare your space and yourself for your massage session, just as you would for a magical ritual. You set your intention and make decisions about how you will implement your Soothing Touch techniques, and then you do them. The final step in the full-body routine—the facial sequence—is the preparation for the third step in a magical ritual: releasing your intention to the universe for manifestation. We'll follow the same generic magical ritual outline you learned earlier, but in our own massage-y way.

Preparing for Your Massage Ritual

A Sacred Massage sequence parallels a magical ritual and, in fact, *is* a ritual—a healing ritual. Just like any ritual, you don't just jump in feetfirst and wing it. (You can, in a pinch, but planning ahead is better.) Physical, mental, and spiritual preparation come first. You plan your ritual from beginning to end in advance, and make sure all the tools you'll need are ready to go near your working altar, which in this case is your massage table. Just like a magical ritual, the Sacred Massage ritual has three parts: intention (your goal for this session), implementation (the full-body massage sequence), and manifestation (releasing your intention to the universe for fulfillment).

Before setting up your massage area for your session, clarify your intention, such as "I will relieve (Buddy's name)'s anxiety and tension." Everything you do in your session will be devoted to implementing that intention and preparing it for manifestation. With your intention in mind, you have a few more things to decide upon before beginning your session.

Deity and Altars

First, choose the healing energy or deity you'd like to include in this Sacred Massage session, and a blessing or mantra associated with that deity, or one that represents their essence. You'll use this mantra at the beginning of your Sacred Massage session to welcome and reinforce that deity's presence and participation. If you wish, you can wear a symbol of your deity, such as a pendant, or place a representation, figurine, or symbol of your healing deity in your massage area. If you prefer a more elaborate tribute to your deity, you could create an altar solely devoted to honoring that deity and welcoming them into your massage session. Include items that would honor and delight that deity, and feel meaningful, inspirational, and genuine to you.

If you'd like a more magically intensive tone for your session, create an "attraction altar" for your massage area to attract the energies and magic you desire. Write your intention on a piece of paper or speak it into an item, and place it on your altar. In addition to attracting certain energies, this attraction altar (as opposed to a working altar where magical work is done) is meant to encourage and reinforce you—the healer. It should inspire peaceful confidence. It should infuse you with "I can do this." For ideas about what to include on your altar, review chapter 3. You can also include any item that is spiritually or magically meaningful to you. Again, an altar can be as simple as a crystal and a candle, or an elaborate magical display.

If you're feeling fancy, you could have a deity altar *and* an attraction altar in your massage space if you wish, or combine them into one beautiful, magical, spiritual arrangement. Let your creativity come out and play. And yes, it's perfectly fine to have more than one altar. I have six of them—and that's just in my massage office!

Spiritual Symbols, Mantras, and Blessings

In addition to the mantra you've chosen to represent your deity, you'll also need to create a personal blessing, from your heart to your Buddy's, such as "I wish you peace and healing" or "May you be refreshed and rejuvenated." Next, choose a symbol, such as the outline of a heart or spiral, or any symbol that's spiritually meaningful to you. You'll invoke this symbol as you finish your Sacred Massage, and channel its energy to your Buddy. Lastly, choose a simple word or blessing, such as "Namaste," "Blessed be," or "Perfect peace" to bring your session to a close.

While your intention may change from person to person (because not every person needs the same thing), your healing deity, mantra, and blessings don't have to. In fact, I find it comforting and reinforcing to use the same cherished ones for all of my clients, because it creates spiritual connectivity between them—they are my precious little unit. They are the only people on Earth who receive that particular sequence of mantras, symbols, and blessings. Also, you may eventually wish to change your deity, symbol, blessings, mantras, and phrases, which is perfectly natural because as you evolve as a healer, the entities and practices you find reinforcing and meaningful may evolve too. Change them, or not. As long as it comes from your heart, it's all good.

Preparing Your Ritual Space

Remember your color magic as you prepare your massage ritual space, and let it reinforce your intention—even the sheets and blankets. Make use of any other magical tools or symbols that would enhance your session.

Before your Buddy arrives, make your massage table comfy and inviting. The sheets should be clean and all wrinkles smoothed away. Fold the top massage sheet back so it's ready for your Buddy to climb on board. With your table set up, look around and make sure your magical massage tools and symbols are in place: oil, holster, blanket, and leg support at the very least, and crystals, figurines, altars, or other magical items if you wish. When you look around, you should feel calm, safe, and peaceful, and also energized and confident. Remove or cover up any items that are contrary to that goal.

Preparing for a Sacred Massage is like planning a dinner party. You decide on the food, decorations, and music before your guests arrive, and make all the preparations in advance. Same thing here. Create a well-prepared, peaceful, welcoming atmosphere that's conducive for all that massage magic to unfold. Just like decorating for a party, how you arrange, adorn, and light a room creates a mood. The mood in your massage area should inspire rest, relaxation, and rejuvenation. Lower the lighting to as dark as you can and still see. If you want music, play it very low, as if trying to lull your Buddy to sleep. Make the area feel like a comforting cocoon of *ahhhhhh*.

Preparing Yourself for Ritual

With everything planned and everything in place, it's time to get yourself ready. Choose your clothing using color magic. Let the colors represent your intention, and wear a pendant that reinforces your connection to your healing deity or represents your magical intention. (Tuck it into the neckline of your shirt if it's so long that it might brush against your Buddy while you work.) A common ritual practice is to bathe beforehand or symbolically bathe by swirling incense or sage smoke around you. Do whichever feels comfortable for you. If your breath is marginal, brush your teeth or chew some mints. Breathing coffee breath (or worse) all over someone's face is gross. Remove all jewelry from your arms and hands, and wash your hands. As you wash your hands, make it a preparatory cleansing ritual, and honor them and thank them for the divine channeling they're about to do.

Just before your session, meditate for a couple minutes and clear your mind of negative or unhelpful thoughts and feelings. Breathe. Devote this upcoming session to serve as a conduit of divine love and compassion, healing, and magical energy. When you feel calm, open, clear, and connected, you're ready to proceed.

Silence Isn't Just Golden—It's Spiritual

There's one more skill to master as you practice your Sacred Massage sequence: silence. Let your Buddy know that you must concentrate and be fully present in your own mind to really absorb this sequence, and conversation is very distracting. However, it's okay for them to let you know if something you're doing hurts or feels uncomfortable.

Limit your conversation to speaking only when absolutely necessary, such as checking in to see if the pressure is okay, letting your Buddy know it's time to turn over, or reminding them to relax if they're "helping" you hold up their arm. Jiggle the arm lightly, and say very softly, "Relax your arm." Nothing more. You need to experience complete, calm, *quiet* focus as you work, and allow the magical energy to flow freely. You must learn how to synchronize with silence.

Sacred Massage Finish

The full-body sequence you learned is typical of any average massage—warmup, actual physical massage work, and a peaceful, gentle finish. That's a wonderful massage all on its own, but it's not a Sacred Massage. A Sacred Massage takes an average massage "next level."

Because you're including divine energy and magical focus, sacred energy runs throughout the session like a current. Even when you're focusing on your hands and what you're doing during the full-body sequence, you're being powered by divine healing magic.

All the Sacred Massage ritual steps before the actual physical Soothing Touch begins are experienced by your Buddy as quiet grounding and centering, breathing, and relaxing. They'll likely be unaware of anything you're doing. Their only job is to relax and receive. Likewise, the finishing blessings following the Soothing Touch sequences are also experienced simply as safe, comforting, quiet time before your Sacred Massage session is done.

Sacred Connection

Remember the facial sequence? While circling the temples, you gradually became more and more aware of yourself, your own body, and your own internal process. Since we're at the temples, it's only natural to commune with deity there. As you share your awareness of yourself and your Buddy, you also reconnect with your deity and channel divine compassion, healing, and relaxation to your Buddy.

As you finish the temples and move your hands to cradle your Buddy's head and breathe, the magical energy comes back online too. You'll shift your awareness even further within yourself—calm, open, and clear for magical energy to flow through you and around you. Invite it in, as if opening a window to let in a cool breeze.

Filled with divine, magical energy, consider what this moment represents. Be present in the moment. Feel the weight of your Buddy's head in your hands, and gaze lovingly upon that sweet, peaceful face. Cradled in your palms is the entire experience of a human lifetime right up to that very moment. Embrace this precious, sacred moment. This person has such complete trust in you, they're allowing you to hold their very existence in your hands. It's as if they've emotionally revisited their own infancy, melting into their mother's arms, completely safe, completely peaceful. Thoroughly *receive* this sacred experience, and recognize it for what it is. It's an honor to be trusted so completely.

Filled with appreciation for being allowed to participate in this sacred moment, you'll bestow your personal blessing to your Buddy in your mind, then trace the spiritual symbol over them, and mentally clear away any residual unwanted energy, and close with a simple word or phrase. You'll complete this entire finishing sequence in your mind. While you're doing all this, your Buddy is simply experiencing a quiet moment in the safety of your hands. For them, it's just a warm, gentle rest before the session ends.

Sacred Massage Outline

In this sequence, we'll fold the full-body sequence into the overall Sacred Massage outline—your Sacred Massage ritual. Rather than rewrite the massage sequences for each area, there's a prompt for "massage sequence for back" and "massage sequence for front," which indicate where to perform the entire full-body massage sequence.

Keep your cheat sheets handy in case you need them, and don't hesitate to look at them if you feel unsure of yourself. We all looked at cheat sheets when we got started. Additionally, write this Sacred Massage ritual outline on something large, like a poster board, and tack it to the wall or prop it up where you can see it at all times. You don't have to write the outline down word for word—just enough to prompt your memory about what to do.

The structure of this Sacred Massage ritual is the same as the magical ritual we learned in Chapter 4; however, we won't use any tools other than your hands and mind, and no sound, other than inhaling and exhaling. In addition to your massage techniques, you'll do this entire massage ritual with thought, breath, and quiet movement only.

Cleanse/Purify: Before beginning, your Buddy already facedown on the table, visualize sweeping any negative or unhelpful energy up and out the door, or scoop it up and blow it out the door like a feather.

Ground and Center: Place your palms side by side on your Buddy's back, over the massage sheet. Inhale from the universe, and exhale into the earth. Feel your connection to the earth, your own body, and then your Buddy. Welcome pure white light through your crown chakra, and receive the divine healing love of the universe. Inhale it, and exhale it out over your Body Buddy. Keep your hands in place.

Cast Your Circle: Visualize white light emerging at the north side of your space, and moving clockwise to create a protective circle of light all the way around you and your Buddy, returning to north to complete the circle. Your magical massage circle is now cast, forming a protective dome of soft white translucent light. Only positive energy may exist within this dome.

Welcome the Energies: Visualize or nod to each direction, beginning at north, and moving clockwise, mentally welcome the directions and energies: "Welcome, energies of the north … comfort and protection," and so on.

Welcome Your Deity: Close your eyes and silently welcome your healing deity into your heart and mind, and your session. Spread your palms apart across your Buddy's back, one to the shoulder, one to the hips, and as you do, mentally spread your deity's mantra or blessing right over your Buddy's back.

Raise Energy: Place a palm on the point of each shoulder, and slowly "rock and walk" the body between your palms, all the way down each side of the body to the feet, and back. You could also lightly brush the entire body with your fingertips.

Recall Your Intention: Slide your palms back to where you started, together on the middle of the back. Recall your intention for this session and let divine presence and magical energy flow through you.

Massage Sequences/Implementation: Do the full-body sequence for the back of the body, then the front. At the facial sequence, while circling the temples, invite your own internal awareness to return as you finish with the head cradled in your hands. Embrace that sacred moment, and open yourself to divine, magical energy. Feel it flowing right through you, infusing your Buddy with pure compassion, relaxation, and healing.

Personal Blessing: Mentally bestow the personal blessing you created for this moment: "May you be well and peaceful, beautiful person."

Bless with Symbol: Still cradling the head, visualize your spiritual symbol and trace it with your chin over your Buddy's body as you inhale. Exhale the symbol, send it out over the body with a push from your chin.

Comb Away Unwanted Energy/Closing: Imagine a big magical comb gliding over the body as you slowly inhale and pull your chin back, catching any residual negative, unhelpful, or unhealthy energy in the comb. Continue inhaling and combing, and swoop the comb up over and behind you, taking the shape of huge gossamer angel wings. Exhale as you visualize the wings dissolving like mist, sprinkling that unwanted energy into the earth to be neutralized. As the wings dissipate, mentally bestow your simple word or phrase for closing your session, such as "Blessed be" or "Namaste."

Manifestation: Continue quietly cradling the head. Mentally release your intention to the universe. Let it fly. The universe receives it, and readies it for manifestation. If you like, acknowledge the release of your intention by mentally commanding, "So mote it be." (This is a traditional Pagan way to end a ritual, and means "May it be so," similar to "Amen" at the end of a prayer.)

Thank the Directions: Still cradling the head, visualize or nod to each direction beginning with north, moving counterclockwise to return to north, and thank the directions: "Thank you, energies of the north," and so on.

Thank Your Deity: Send thoughts of gratitude to your healing deity: "Thank you, Kuan Yin."

Uncast Your Circle: Beginning at north, visualize the white circle of light and its translucent dome dissolving as you turn your attention to each direction, counterclockwise, returning to north. Your magical circle is dissolved, and you and your Buddy now return to "reality."

Shoulder Squeeze: Softly, slowly, slide your hands out from under the head, and gently slide your palms out over the top of each shoulder, your fingers draping gently over the points of the shoulders. Give their shoulders a very subtle, loving squeeze.

Ending the Session

Although you've returned to reality after the shoulder squeeze, your Buddy may need some time to come back. They might even be sound asleep and not notice your cue that the session is over. If time isn't an issue, just quietly leave the room and let them sleep. If waking them up is necessary, do not startle them from this deeply relaxed state. Coax them back to consciousness gently by whispering their name, and lightly touching their head or shoulder.

Quietly leave the room or area, so they can get dressed. Meanwhile, lovingly and appreciatively wash your hands in cool water, and thank these amazing magical tools for their service. In a magical ritual, a celebration usually follows in the form of chatting and refreshments, and you can do the same with your Buddy if you wish.

You Did It!

Congratulations on completing your first Sacred Massage! Don't worry if it felt awkward, don't worry if you missed a step or got lost and had to go back, don't worry if it seemed like a whole lot to think about and you fear you'll be using your cheat sheets forever. (Trust me, you won't!)

This is only your first dance rehearsal. You just walked through all the steps of the entire dance. Sure, there are lots of halts and do-overs, stumbles and missteps, and it may feel clumsy and discombobulated now. But once a dancer steps on stage, the dance is fluid and gorgeous. The point is—it doesn't start that way! Whether a dance routine or Sacred

Massage, it's all about practice, practice, practice. Dancers keep practicing until the whole dance just flows from their spirit. It will be the same for you, and the good news is—your feet won't hurt nearly as much!

Taking a Different Position

We've learned our various massage sequences so far with the assumption that your Buddy is lying on a massage table, mainly to have a consistent, coherent conversation. If your loved one is unable to lie on a massage table and will need to be in a different position, or if you don't yet have a table, now we'll talk about how to deal with these situations.

We also initially learned massage sequences in segments. Think of these segments as components that you can add to or remove from the massage session you tailor to your loved one. Although you know how to do a full-body massage, it isn't necessary to do that entire sequence in order to do a Sacred Massage. You can pick and choose the components for *your* Sacred Massage session. If your loved one must be in a different position for your session, such as sitting in a chair, some of the sequences you learned will work in that position, and some won't. Don't frustrate yourself and attempt to do all the segments you learned—figure out which ones *will* work, and customize the sequences for your loved one.

Also, your loved one may not even *want* you to do all of those segments. Not everyone wants a full-body relaxation massage. Some people just want their back, shoulders, and neck worked on. Others would really just love a long, luxurious foot massage. Other people have an injury they'd like you to focus upon or stay away from. Whatever your loved one wants—give it to them. Getting a Sacred Massage—or any massage for that matter—isn't like being told, "Eat your broccoli, young lady," or "Clean your plate" when you're a kid at the dinner table. Nope. Your loved one gets to decide what they want, and you tailor your Soothing Touch techniques and sequences to accommodate it. Trust your loved one enough to know what they want, and proceed from there, without argument. There's no ego in Sacred Massage. It's all about your loved one, and what *they* need and want.

If your loved one prefers a not-so-full-body massage, or must sit or lie in a position other than how we learned the sequences, customize your massage sequences to suit their needs or desires. Maybe they don't want you to work on their feet or their face. That's okay. Drop those sequences from your massage routine. If all you can work on is Grandpa's neck and shoulders, replace the back and front of the body sequences in the Sacred Massage outline with "Grandpa's sequence"—the one you create. If the only Soothing Touch you can provide to your loved one is to gently place your palms on their body, hold their hand, and lovingly massage their scalp, then *that* is the massage sequence for your loved one's Sacred Massage. Make the massage fit the loved one, not vice versa.

Once you create your own sequences just for your loved one, you can rewrite the Sacred Massage outline and replace "sequences for back and front of the body" with your new sequences. Everything else in the Sacred Massage outline remains the same.

Maybe you or your loved one like a sequence, but not a particular tool. Ditch it. You don't have to use the tools or techniques I shared, or in the order I shared them—only the ones you want. The methods we covered are but a small fraction of the many massage tools and techniques there are, and all it takes is a little googling to discover many, many more. Blend those in with the tools and techniques you like, and really make those massage sequences your own.

Adapting Sacred Massage for Other Positions, Situations, and Circumstances

If your loved one can't comfortably lie on their stomach and/or back, there are other options. If you get stumped by a restriction, you'll have to find a creative solution. You may have to reinvent your entire approach to Sacred Massage. That's okay. My outline isn't an edict. Shape your Sacred Massage to suit your loved one, and their situation. There's not a "right or wrong" way to do this—there's only the way that works for you and your loved one. Let's explore some alternatives to lying on the stomach and back.

Reclining Position

Some people aren't able to lie on their backs at all. One of my clients had "ankylosing spondylosis," which made his spine curve into a hunch, the vertebrae fused in that position by the disease. It was physically impossible for him to lie flat on his back so I could work on his neck and shoulders. However, he could lean back in a reclining position onto some fluffy pillows, and that worked just fine.

A reclining position works great for the neck and shoulders, as well as the pecs, scalp, ears, jaws, face, arms, hands, and front of the legs and feet. You can work on these areas the same way you learned, making accommodations for your own body being in a different position. You may have to adjust the angle of your hands, and use muscle power rather than body weight to increase pressure. To add some extra comfort in a reclining position, place a pillow, rolled towel, or bolster under the knees. To work on the back of the body, if your loved one is unable to lie flat or can't lie on their stomach, position them on their side.

If your loved one must remain in a hospital bed, you may be able to lift the head of the bed and stand behind it to access the pecs, shoulders, neck, and head. Hands, arms, the front of the legs, and feet are also easily accessible if your loved one is in a hospital bed. Lying on the stomach in a hospital bed may not be comfortable, or even possible, so position your loved one on their side to access the back and back of the legs.

Side-lying Massage

You'll need three bed-sized pillows to do a side-lying massage. One goes between the knees to relieve stress on the knees and hips. One goes under the head and neck to keep the cervical spine straight and prevent the head from flopping down sideways. The third goes right against their chest and tummy, relieving stress on the shoulder and arm that are on top, and giving them something comforting to hug.

For side-lying massage, you'll need to change the sequence up a bit. You'll do one entire side of the body—neck to toes—on one side, and then turn over and do the entire other side, rather than repeating sequences on each side for each sequence as we did while learning. This includes the back and back of the shoulders—one half while lying on one side, the other half while lying on the other.

When it's time to turn over, pull all the pillows out, assist your loved one to turn onto the other side, and replace all the pillows. The side-lying position works for those who can't lie on their stomachs or backs for any reason, such as pregnancy, health condition, or following surgery or an injury.

You can do most of the moves for the front and back of the body in a side-lying position; however, you'll have to adjust the angle of your hands and arms. You also won't be able to use your body weight to increase pressure, and will have to use your muscles.

Before practicing a side-lying massage on your Body Buddy, google "side-lying massage" and watch some videos to get some ideas for this position.

Propping for Pain or Stiffness

You prop the body to place any limb or area into a neutral position. Someone with arthritis, joint issues, back pain, or recent surgery or injury typically might need to have something propped. Massage bolsters are great because they slide easily in and out from under the sheet or body, and come in all shapes and sizes; however, you can get by just fine with things you have around the house.

Hand towels are so versatile. They can be folded to just the right depth to prop under that sore spot and get it into a neutral position, such as under the shoulder if your loved one has chronic shoulder pain. A hand towel rolled longways can be placed under the neck while your loved one is lying faceup to support the cervical spine and allow it to relax.

If knee pain is an issue while lying facedown, a folded hand towel above and below the knee can provide relief. If lower back pain is an issue, prop the knees with a rolled-up bath towel or pillow(s) when your loved one is lying faceup. Your loved one may prefer their entire lower legs to be propped while faceup, which can easily be done with pillows. Those with circulation issues in the legs or swelling in the feet or ankles may also appreciate having their lower legs propped while faceup.

Bath-sized towels also come in handy. Besides using a rolled towel under the knees, they can provide relief for large-breasted women or someone with tender breasts. The towel is placed above the breasts, supporting under the upper pectorals, not on the breast tissue.

Working Over Clothing

If your loved one will remain clothed during your session, you'll have to limit yourself to those manual tools and techniques that don't require oil to do long, gliding moves. You could still glide a Snowplow or Steamroller over the clothing on the back, but you'll have to work lightly because the friction from the clothing will irritate your skin. For deeper work, you'll have to rely on pressing, kneading, squeezing, and leaning, rather than gliding and sliding. You can lean your body weight into the heels of your hands, the flats of your Irons, or your Power Points, and your Duckbill will still work well over clothing. You can still do gentle stretches if your loved one's clothing is stretchy. You can still jiggle or "rock and roll" any limb or the whole body to loosen them up, and you can still give a pretty darn good foot massage right over socks—squeezing, pressing, and kneading the sole and top of the foot, and gently pulling and stretching the toes.

When your loved one prefers to remain clothed, you should still have access to the hands, neck, jaw, ears, face, and scalp, and can work on these areas just as you learned.

Seated/Chair Massage

Chair massage comes in handy for someone who prefers to remain clothed as well as for someone who doesn't like or want to lie down for their massage. There are very comfortable massage chairs available, or you can mimic this position by placing a stool next to a table or counter, and having your Buddy sit on it, facing the counter. They can fold their arms on the counter, and rest their forehead on their folded arms. Whether they're in a massage chair or sitting next to a counter, you're pretty much limited to working on the arms, hands, back, shoulders, neck, ears, jaw, and scalp, and only able to use oil on whatever skin is exposed.

Chair massage is its own animal, and quite different from working on a table. Not only are the techniques limited, but there's the added difficulty of working over clothing, with the same restrictions—pressing, kneading, squeezing, and leaning, rather than gliding and sliding. You can do a streamroller from the tops of the shoulders, sliding down the trapezius, but it'll make your elbow raw pretty quick. You can also lean your Steamroller onto the top of the shoulder and hold, which will provide some relief to tight shoulders.

For chair/seated massage, rock and jiggle the shoulders, back, and arms to warm them up, and slide your palms over them. Pressing with your Irons, heels of your hand, or thumbs will also provide relief; however, you'll have to lift and move your hands from spot to spot rather than glide them.

When working on the back in chair massage, make use of gravity and the angle of the back to slide or walk your fists from the shoulder to the iliac crest alongside the spine, in the muscle, not on the spine. Leaning the heels of your hands at the top of the lumbar spine and pressing them down to the iliac crest is a great move for chair/seated massage, and that good old classic massage move—the double shoulder kneading—will work for this position.

If your loved one is wearing a sleeveless shirt, you can still do the same arm sequences that you already learned, in this new position. You'll be glad you tried pinning the wrist between your upper arm and rib cage when you did chair massage, because it leaves both your hands free to knead, slide, and squeeze. If your loved one is wearing long sleeves, your Duckbill can make slow, deep "bites" all along the forearm, and on over the upper arm. Your Duck will have to open wide, and you may need both of them at once to squeeze the upper arm. Finish the arms by sliding your palms down the length of the arm to hold the hand, and then continue with the same hand sequences you already learned. Finish with a firm but gentle squeeze on the hand, and a gentle arm stretch.

The sequence for the back of the neck and scalp are the same in chair massage, and many of the techniques for the upper back will work. Finish by brushing your fingers all over the areas you massaged, ending at the tops of the shoulders with a nice, loving squeeze, or finish with some luxurious scalp scratching.

You'll need to practice chair massage on your Buddy to get the hang of chair/seated massage, and anyone else who'd like a free on-the-spot shoulder and neck massage. You don't need any oil, and can just flip an office chair sideways, and use a desk to prop the arms and head. You'll be the most popular person in your office.

As with side-lying massage, I strongly recommend you watch some chair massage videos to see how it goes, and which tools and techniques work best. Getting a chair massage yourself will also inspire some ideas.

If your loved one must remain in a chair or wheelchair, again, you'll only be able to work on the areas you have access to, and most will be over clothing. Focus on those areas you can reach, such as the hands, arms, upper shoulders, neck, head, front of thighs, and lower leg and feet, and select the tools and techniques that will still work for this situation.

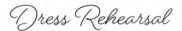

Dress Rehearsal

Take some time to really analyze your loved one's needs, including any physical condition they have, clothing they might wear, and what position they might be in—sitting or lying. If you don't have a massage table or chair, or neither of those is appropriate, you'll need to decide where you'll work: on the floor, in a bed or chair, or with a wheelchair. Visualize the entire scenario in your mind—walk through it from beginning to end, noting every possible concern or issue you can imagine. From this scenario, create massage sequences for each area you can work on, and substitute them for the full-body sequences in the Sacred Massage outline.

Before actually working on your loved one, practice your entire customized sequence on your Buddy, using the exact same restrictions or changes. Have your Buddy sit or lie in the position your loved one will be in, and treat it like a real dress rehearsal—make everything just as it will be with your loved one, including propping and working over clothing. This will provide on-the-spot information about whether or not you need to tweak your sequence to make it flow more smoothly. You may discover that you need to improvise and experiment, or use a different tool or technique. You may need to drop something from your special sequence entirely. Ask your Buddy for feedback—what felt great, and what still needs adjusting.

It Will Still Be Sacred

No matter what position or situation you must accommodate to provide massage to your loved one, you can still create a Sacred Massage experience. Your warm, loving compassion, and genuine concern for your loved one's health and welfare, will fill in all the gaps. Even if all you can do is gently hold a hand and lovingly stroke the hair, you can still do the complete Sacred Massage ritual, channel divine love and compassion, and infuse the entire process with magical intention. It's your *touch*, not the technique, that ultimately makes a massage experience sacred.

My Magical Blend

You may have noticed that I don't stick to one magical or spiritual tradition for Sacred Massage (or anything else, for that matter). I'm a magical and spiritual hunter-gatherer. I explore all sorts of paths and practices, and collect things that I find inspirational, useful, and valuable to create my own unique divine, magical practices. My massage practice includes devotion to a Buddhist deity, Reiki imagery, magical meditation and visualization, angel imagery, and traditional Pagan blessings and practices. My spiritual, magical conglomeration might give a purist heartburn, but I'm a "Garden-Variety Pagan," and "eclectic" is how I roll. My spiritual and magical practices are completely genuine, completely unique, completely me. I invite you to do the same, and be genuinely, completely, uniquely *you*. Unless you're firmly committed to a particular spiritual practice or path, try things out as you evolve as a healer, and create your own divine, magical Sacred Massage sequences.

Think of what I've shared with you not as a framework, but as a springboard for your own magical massage work. You can keep using what you've learned in this book, or change it up to suit your own spiritual, magical, or divine preferences. Make this massage practice your own, not my costume that you wear for awhile. This is *your* Sacred Massage practice—you make the rules, you create the template. You could work just with healing pink light if you want, or the whole shebang and invite the all-encompassing God/universe/Spirit—or anything in between, and any combination thereof. You can change my words or imagery if something else feels better to you—maybe a gentle breeze rather than a huge comb removing that unwanted energy clearing, and sending it off onto the winds rather than down to the earth. Ultimately, it matters less which specific spiritual and magical techniques you use than it does that everything you do feels genuine, comfortable, and meaningful to you. There's no pretending in magic, or in Sacred Massage.

Conclusion

You Have Everything You Need

Here we are, at the end of our Sacred Massage journey together. From here, you'll move forward and carve your own path, and take my template and mold it into your own. You have everything you need to create a Sacred Massage experience for your loved one. You've learned a little about what they teach you in massage school, and a whole lot about what they don't.

Although you have some really great tools in your massage toolbox, clearly we didn't cover every massage tool or technique that you would in massage school, or all the intermediate and advanced skills offered in continuing education classes. Is there more to learn? Oh heavens, yes.

Right now, you've got a nice, shiny new beginner's box of crayons, with the eight basic colors. You can create a perfectly lovely picture with just these, and this might be all you or your loved one want or need. If you and your loved one are happy, that's great. Keep doing what you do. However, as you continue forward, you may start yearning for the deluxe sixty-four-color crayon box. You'll discover all those wonderful new colors by watching massage videos, reading massage books, taking classes, and most important of all, getting lots of massage for yourself. Learning by experiencing is invaluable.

But maybe you want even *more*.

You may get that big box of crayons and create some amazing works of art, but ultimately decide that what you really desire is the ultimate, super-duper-deluxe set of 152 crayons, with the cool plastic caddy and built-in sharpener! If you want it, go for it! If your Sacred Massage experience whets your appetite to go further, why not go to massage school for formal training? It's a wonderful profession, based in the healing industry, with all sorts of options and flexibility, from working with a chiropractic or medical team, to working in a spa, to setting out on your own and building your own practice.

If you want to bring your Soothing Touch next level and go pro, get out and explore all the options for making it happen. Find out if there's a school near you, and what's involved in getting a professional massage practitioner's certificate. And that's only the start of all the techniques and modalities you'll discover in continuing education and specialized classes. There's so much to learn. Just imagine what your Soothing Touch sequences might become! Just imagine what *you* might become! Anything and everything is possible when you're motivated by love, compassion, and healing.

As for you and I, for now, we must part.

Hail and farewell, you healer, you!

Resources

Here are a few tips to find supplies and resources you might need for massage:

Supplies
(tables, sheets, oil, tools)

Bodywork Mall: *https://www.bodyworkmall.com*
EarthLite: *https://www.earthlite.com*
Massage Warehouse: https://www.massagewarehouse.com

Anatomy
(muscles, skeleton, nervous system, organs)

Healthline: https://www.healthline.com/human-body-maps
Innerbody Research: https://www.innerbody.com/htm/body.html

Information
(education, licensing, finding massage therapists)

American Massage Therapy Association: https://www.amtamassage.org
Associated Bodywork & Massage Professionals: https://www.abmp.com
Massage Therapy License.org: https://www.massagetherapylicense.org

Professional Massage Training

If you're interested in a professional career in massage therapy, here are a few things to consider:

Licensing and Requirements

Massage licensing and certification differ from state to state, county to county, and city to city. Some allow you to work professionally with a basic 100-hour certificate, others may require a 500-hour certificate, and still others may require a 1,000-hour certificate. Some areas require passage of the Massage and Bodywork Licensing Examination (MBLEx), and others do not. Those who use the title of "massage therapist" are required to pass the exam in most states in the US. However, areas may allow you to use the title of "massage practitioner" if you've taken the required schooling but have not taken the exam.

In California, for example, the state doesn't conduct massage certification. A private, non-profit corporation issues certifications for massage professionals that meet certain requirements; however, the state doesn't actually require those "requirements." The state does require you to submit fingerprints and pass a criminal background check. You'll have to find out what your own state requires, as well as your county and city. If you want to have a home office, you'll need to check with your local government office to see what is required, and will likely need to apply for a business license.

Private Practice vs. Employee

One of the main decisions about pursuing a career in massage therapy is whether to have your own private practice or to work for a chiropractor or health facility, or at a spa or gym. The basic decision is autonomy vs. steady income and benefits.

The benefits of private practice are that you set your own wages, make your own hours, and choose your clients. However, you must also pay all the costs of maintaining an office and running a business. This allows you to write off these costs against your income when paying your federal income tax, and you will be responsible for documenting these costs and expenses.

Another consideration for private practice is that there are no benefits, unless you have the willpower to create a savings account to cover illnesses, vacations, and retirement. If you get sick, injured, or go on vacation, your income stops. Also, because you are not receiving a paycheck from an employer, it will be up to you to cover your federal and state taxes. If you want to contribute to your Social Security fund or retirement, you'll need to arrange for that yourself.

If you work for someone else, you'll likely get an hourly wage or flat fee for each massage, but may not get to pick your schedule or your clients. You may be required to do multiple appointments, back to back, with little time for a break in between. Because you are an employee, you may be entitled to sick leave and vacation pay, as well as healthcare benefits and retirement—it differs from employer to employer. As an employee, your federal and state income tax and Social Security will likely be deducted from your paycheck.

Available Training

You can go to a private certified massage school or a community college to get your massage education. A private school may cost substantially more than community college. Visit the education options in your area to find out what is involved to get your certificate and what it costs, and also to get a gut feel for the place to see if you like it. You can take additional continuing education after getting your certificate, in whatever modality or skill interests you.

Talk with Other Massage Therapists

One of the best ways to find out about a career is to talk to others already in that line of work. Make massage appointments, and ask the therapist where they got their training and how they like their job. Most are happy to talk about their career path. Make appointments with therapists that specialize in different modalities so you can experience how they differ and what they do. This means getting *lots* of massage. The more, the better. I know it's tough, but yet, we must just sally forth and endure.

Strength and Stamina

Another consideration before pursuing massage therapy as a career is your own strength and stamina. Massage is a physically demanding profession, and requires you to be on your feet a lot. Even if you practice good body mechanics and posture, it can strain your back, arms, and hands over time. You also must be able to shelve your emotions if you're having a bad day—take a deep breath, ground and center, and walk into that room and be one hundred percent peaceful and present. And you must be just as peaceful and present for the last person you see as you were for the first. You can't start out at one hundred percent and peter out over the day and give your last client only ten percent. Every client gets one hundred percent, just as if they were your first appointment of the day. Massage requires both physical and emotional stamina.

Is Massage Your New Path?

Although there are some requirements and considerations to take into account before embarking on a massage career, and you must invest some time and money, this can be a rewarding career. Massage is a beautiful, peaceful, fulfilling profession, and if you have a love of healing and helping people live more comfortably and completely, this career may suit you. And it's one of those jobs that can't be outsourced. You'll never have to worry about your job being sent overseas.

If this book and the things you've learned here have you wondering, "What if …" then you owe it to yourself to find out. Curiosity is a wonderful thing. It leads you to doors you never considered opening before.

Appendix

Cheat Sheets

Here are all of the Cheat Sheets mentioned throughout the book, in one handy spot. They are listed in the order they would be performed in a full-body massage.

Back of the Body

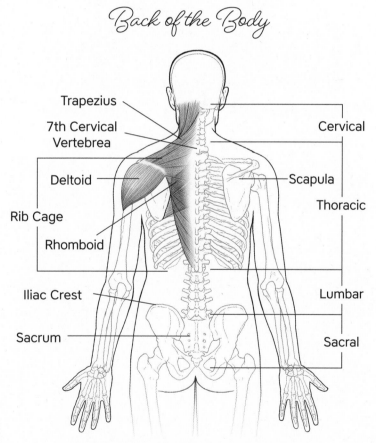

FIGURE 13: BACK, SPINE, AND MUSCLES

Back: "Rock and walk" the whole body; glide and slide; Snowplow; Iron; Rake; Steamroller, one arm; Steamroller, two arms; Powerpoint on trapezius; palm slide on lower back; thumbs on lower back; Scraper on lower back; palm slide on lower back, ending at shoulder.

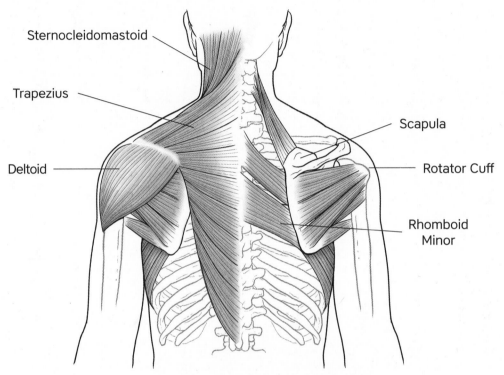

Sternocleidomastoid

Trapezius

Deltoid

Scapula

Rotator Cuff

Rhomboid Minor

FIGURE 14: BACK OF SHOULDERS, SCAPULA, AND NECK

Shoulders and Scapula: Knead both shoulders; Rake one shoulder with both hands, then the other; make a Chicken Wing; press thumb under scapula; use tools of your choice on trapezius; Steamroll circles around scapula.

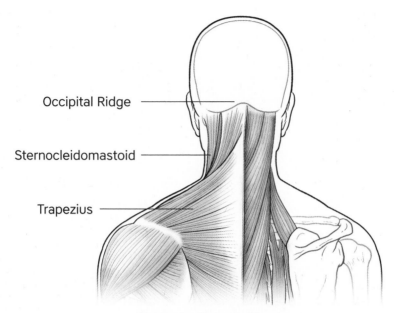

Occipital Ridge

Sternocleidomastoid

Trapezius

Figure 15: Back of Neck

Neck: Duckbill the neck; knead, squeeze, and slide; repeat on other side; slide heels of hands from neck to shoulder; slide Irons from neck to shoulder; gentle scalp scratch.

All Together Now: Back/Shoulders/Neck: Because the muscles of the back, shoulders, and neck work in concert, you'll flow right from the back sequence into the shoulders, scapulae, and neck.

Finishing the Back of the Upper Body: Stand at the head of the table, facing the feet. Slide both palms side by side simultaneously alongside the spine to the hips, swoop outwards to circle over the hips, and reconnect on each side of the spine. Drag relaxed palms slowly back like heavy, wet washcloths. At the top of the back, swoop palms outward over each scapula, as you did the hips. Reconnect palms side by side on each side of the spine, and repeat this "doggy bone" pattern. On the last pass, swipe palms up the back of the neck, then press down the top of each shoulder simultaneously, finishing with one palm on the point of each shoulder. Pull the massage sheet up to cover the back.

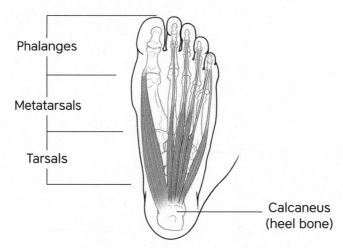

Figure 16: Bottom of Foot/Sole

Foot (sole): Iron sole; Iron circles on sole; thumb circles on sole; squeeze and squish heel; brush sole and toes.

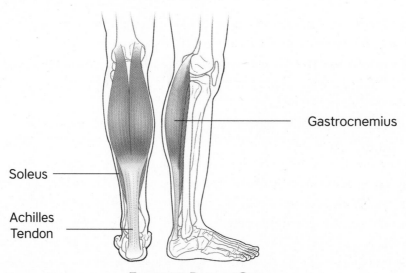

Figure 17: Back of Calf

Calf (back): Jiggle and knead; palm slides on both sides of gastroc; Iron on both sides; Steamroll both sides; knead both heads of gastroc at once; Duckbill slides on Achilles tendon; palm slides up and then down all the way over sole.

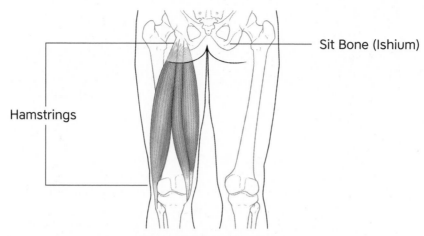

FIGURE 18: BACK OF THIGH

Thigh (back): Jiggle and rock; knead, soften, and warm; palm slides; Iron; Steamroll; knead and slide; sweep over entire leg.

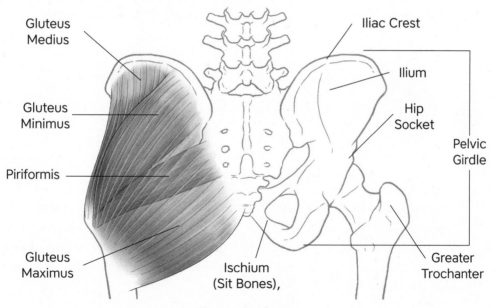

FIGURE 19: GLUTES

Glutes: Rock glutes with heels of hands; Iron curved gutter between lower ilium and greater trochanter; Iron glutes with both hands to "wipe the bowl"; walk Irons to "punch the dough"; press and hold thumb on The Spot; lean Powerpoint into The Spot; walk Irons over glutes.

Finishing the Back of the Lower Body: Combine the cheat sheets for the foot, calf, thigh and glutes into one segment. Do the combined sequence in order (foot, calf, thigh, glutes) on one leg, then repeat on the other leg. Finish the entire back of the leg as you finished the thigh: sweep your palms up from the sole to just under the butt, and sweep back down, brushing over the toes.

Front of the Body

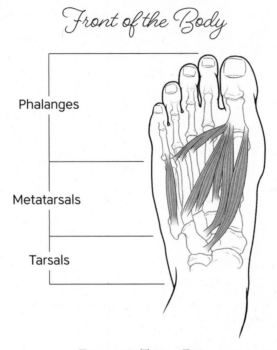

FIGURE 20: TOP OF FOOT

Foot (top): Double Duckbill toothpaste squeeze; loosen foot in figure eight; more toothpaste squeezes; knuckle grind sole; thumb presses on arch; slide down foot over toes, press toes toward sole, stretch top of foot; press ball toward top of foot while pulling on heel, stretch Achilles tendon; more double Duckbill squeezes; brush over toes.

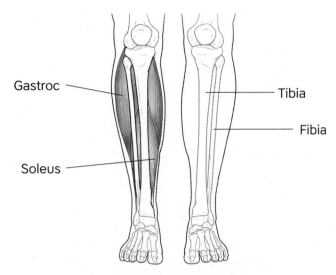

FIGURE 21: FRONT LOWER LEG

Lower Leg (front): Duckbill slides; Duckbill circles; palm slides up both sides of shin, palm pulls underneath gastroc; Achilles tendon stretch; slide over feet, brush toes.

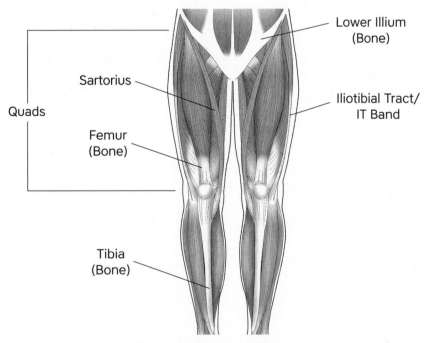

FIGURE 22: FRONT OF THIGH

Thigh (front): Palm slide warmup; Duckbill kneading; "wipe the car" in figure eights; palm slides over quads; steamroll quads; Iron IT band; palm slides over quads; palm slides over length of leg; brush toes.

Finishing the Front of the Lower Body: Combine the sequences for the foot, lower leg, and thigh and perform on the front of one leg, then the other. Finish by sweeping up gently from the top of the foot and over the thigh, and back down again.

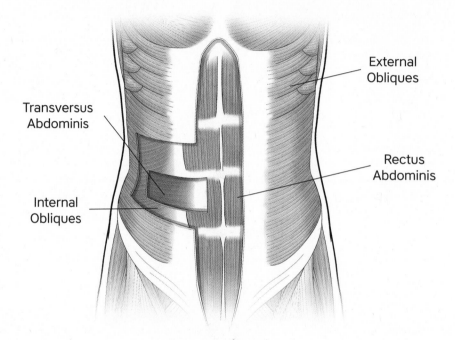

FIGURE 23: STOMACH

Stomach: Spread oil, place palms, hold, breathe; back-and-forth palm slides; waistline pulls; palm circles around belly button; slide palms apart and stretch.

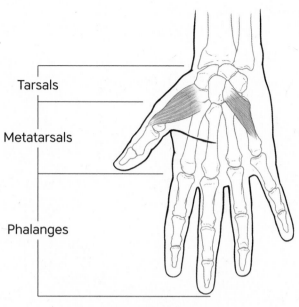

Tarsals

Metatarsals

Phalanges

FIGURE 24: HAND

Hand: Squeeze and slide between metacarpals; squeeze and squish length of each finger and thumb; squeeze and squish little finger muscles; pinch web, press and hold; thumb circles on palm.

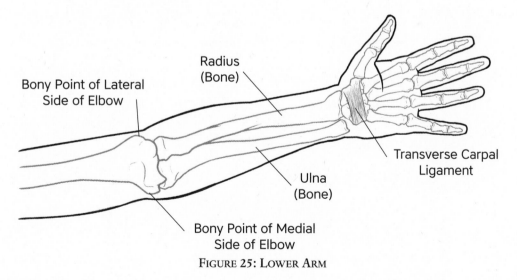

Bony Point of Lateral
Side of Elbow

Radius
(Bone)

Transverse Carpal
Ligament

Ulna
(Bone)

Bony Point of Medial
Side of Elbow

FIGURE 25: LOWER ARM

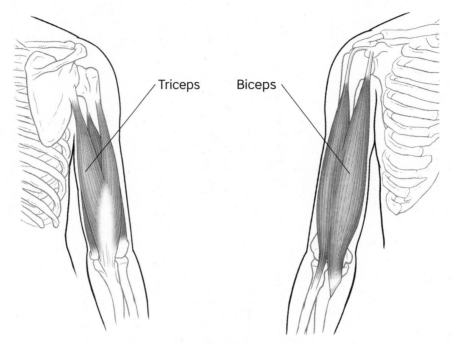

Triceps   Biceps

FIGURE 26: UPPER ARM

Arm: Duckbill bites on forearm; Duckbill forearm slides with one hand and then the other; Duckbill forearm slides with alternating hands; heel slides length of forearm; palm slides; gently pull hand; spread oil on upper arm; pin upper arm; big Duckbill slides; Duckbill kneading; deltoid presses; knead deltoid; palm slides along entire arm; gently pull hand.

Hand and Arm Together: Move from the hand directly to the forearm and upper arm, then switch sides to repeat on the other hand and arm.

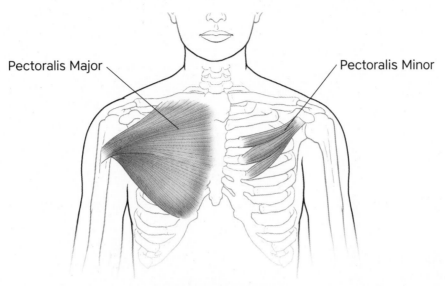

Figure 27: Pectorals

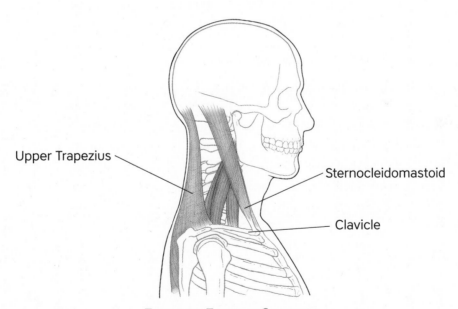

Figure 28: Front of Shoulder

Pectorals and Shoulders: Palm slides across pectorals; Iron pectorals; squeeze pectorals below armpits; palm slides out over pectorals and deltoids, and up shoulder tops, ending in Duckbill on shoulders; Duckbill kneads on shoulders; heel slides along shoulder tops; Iron shoulder tops; Iron "marching" on shoulder tops; deep Duckbill kneads; palm slides from underneath back to shoulders, and outward along shoulder tops; palm slides over pectorals and deltoids, over top of shoulder and up sides of neck, stopping at head.

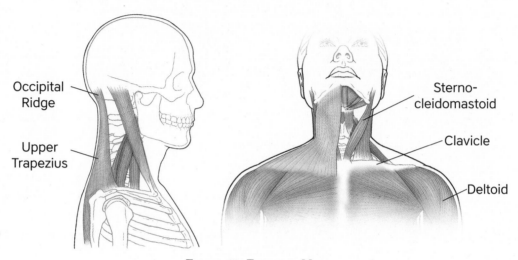

Occipital Ridge

Upper Trapezius

Sterno-cleidomastoid

Clavicle

Deltoid

FIGURE 29: FRONT OF NECK

Neck: Massage occipital ridge; fingertip circles on both sides of neck; turn head and apply oil; circles over triangle; fingers, Scraper, Iron, and knuckles along top of shoulder and back of neck; knead and smoosh neck; knead and smoosh top of shoulder; soft knuckle slides on side of neck, then include top of shoulder; heel slides from side of neck down over top of shoulder; Iron from side of neck down over top of shoulder; switch hands; finish by swooping over pecs, deltoids, shoulders, and up neck, stopping to cradle head in palms.

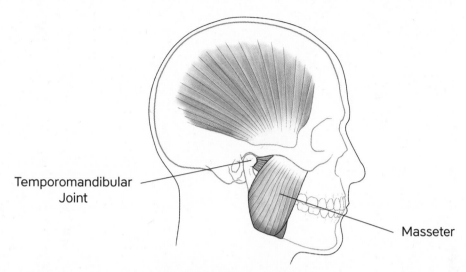

Temporomandibular Joint

Masseter

Figure 30: Jaw and Scalp

Scalp and Ears: Finger slides over occipital ridge; slide fingers back and forth under head; all-over fingertip massage; thumb slides on top of head; press scalp over skull; scratch; drag through hair; squeeze circles on earlobes; pull lobes; circle squeezes on outer ear curls; pull ears away from head; smooshy squeeze.

Jaw and Face: Press circles over masseter, first one way, then the other; scrape from masseter to bottom corner of jaw; slide palms along jawline; press light circles in center of cheeks; slide chin in circles; forehead massage; circle temples while reconnecting to your breath, body, and Spirit; slide hands under head to cradle it; breathe, rest, and connect.

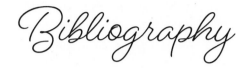

Bibliography

Books

Beck, Mark E. *Theory & Practice of Therapeutic Massage*. Fifth Edition. Clifton Park, NY: Milady, 2010.

Changaris, Michael. *Touch: The Neurobiology of Health, Healing, and Human Connection*. Mendocino, California: LifeRhythm and Core Evaluation Publications, 2015.

DeAngelo, Debra. *Pagan Curious: A Beginner's Guide to Nature, Magic & Spirituality*. Woodbury, MN: Llewellyn Publications, 2022.

Janson, Eva Rudy. *The Book of Buddhas: Ritual Symbolism Used on Buddhist Statuary and Ritual Objects*. Haarlem, Holland: Binkey Kok Publications, 2006.

Monaghan, Patricia. *Encyclopedia of Goddesses & Heroines*. Novato, CA: New World Library, 2014.

Ortner, Nick. *The Tapping Solution: A Revolutionary System for Stress-Free Living*. Carlsbad, CA: Hay House Publications, 2013.

Penczak, Christopher. *Magick of Reiki: Focused Energy for Healing, Ritual & Spiritual Development*. Woodbury, MN: Llewellyn Publications, 2007.

RavenWolf, Silver. *Angels: Companions in Magick*. Woodbury, MN: Llewellyn Publications, 2019 (original edition, 1996).

Schenker, Daniela. *Kuan Yin: Accessing the Power of the Divine Feminine*. Boulder, CO: Sounds True, 2007.

Weber, Courtney. *Brigid: History, Mystery, and Magick of the Celtic Goddess*. San Francisco, CA: Red Wheel/Weiser LLC, 2015.

Yrizarry, Shannon. *Modern Guide to Meditation Beads*. Woodbury, MN: Llewellyn Publications, 2020.

Online

Adams, Rose; Barb White, and Cynthia Beckett. "The Effects of Massage Therapy on Pain Management in the Acute Care Setting." National Center for Biotechnology Information. March 17, 2010. https://www.ncbi.nlm.nih.gov/pmc/articles/PMC3091428/.

American Association of Neurological Surgeons. "Anatomy of the Spine and Peripheral Nervous System." Accessed March 29, 2022. AANS.org. https://www.aans.org/en/Patients/Neurosurgical-Conditions-and-Treatments/Anatomy-of-the-Spine-and-Peripheral-Nervous-System.

Associated Bodywork & Massage Professionals (ABMP). "Find a Massage Therapist or Bodyworker." Accessed November 5, 2021. https://www.massagetherapy.com/glossary.

Atlantic Religion. "Sirona—Another Syncretic Guise of the Celtic 'Great Goddess'." August 29, 2014. The Atlantic Religion. https://atlanticreligion.com/2014/08/29/sirona-another-syncretic-guise-of-the-celtic-great-goddess/.

Bach, Marilyn. "What Does the Research Say?" University of Minnesota. Accessed October 20, 2021. https://www.takingcharge.csh.umn.edu/explore-healing-practices/healing-touch/what-does-research-say.

Brazier, Yvette. "Health Benefits of Basil." MedicalNewsToday.com. December 16, 2019. https://www.medicalnewstoday.com/articles/266425.

Cartwright, Mark. "Asclepius." WorldHistory.org. June 20, 2013. https://www.worldhistory.org/Asclepius/.

Catlin, Ann. "The Role of Massage Therapy in Dementia Care." Massage Today. March 16, 2015. https://www.massagetoday.com/articles/15057/The-Role-of-Massage-Therapy-in-Dementia-Care.

Cerritelli, Francesco; Piero Chiacchiaretta, Francesco Gambi, Antonio Ferretti. "Effect of Continuous Touch on Brain Functional Connectivity is Modified by the Operator's Attention." Frontiers in Human Neuroscience. July 20, 2017. https://www.frontiersin.org/articles/10.3389/fnhum.2017.00368/full.

Coan, James Q.; Hillary S. Schaefer, Richard J. Davidson. "Lending a hand: social regulation of the neural response to threat." National Library of Medicine. December 2006. https://pubmed.ncbi.nlm.nih.gov/17201784/.

Creveling, Mallory. "The Healing Power of Touch May Be the Missing Link." The Well. Accessed October 20, 2021. https://www.the-well.com/editorial/the-healing-power-of-touch.

Dimancea, Vlad. "Cho Ku Rei: Explore The Untapped Potential of A Versatile Reiki Symbol." ReikiScoop. January 3, 2022. https://reikiscoop.com/cho-ku-rei-reiki-symbol/.

Dobson, Roger. "How the Power of Touch Reduces Pain and Even Fights Disease." Independent. October 23, 2011. https://www.independent.co.uk/life-style/health-and-families/health-news/how-the-power-of-touch-reduces-pain-and-even-fights-disease-419462.html.

Durand, Marcella. "Massage Therapy for Seniors." American Massage Therapy Association. August 1, 2020. https://www.amtamassage.org/publications/massage-therapy-journal/massage-for-elderly/.

Field, Tiffany. "Massage Therapy Research Review." National Center for Biotechnology Information. June 12, 2017. https://www.ncbi.nlm.nih.gov/pmc/articles/PMC5467308/.

Florida Academy. "The History of Massage Therapy: 5,000 Years of Relaxation and Pain Relief. May 17, 2019. https://florida-academy.edu/history-of-massage-therapy/.

Flowers, Rebecca. "This is What Sensory Processing Disorder Feels Like to People With Autism." Massage Magazine. April 17, 2018. https://www.massagemag.com/sensory-processing-disorder-autism-cst-88859/.

Goddess Gift. "Yemaya: Goddess of the Ocean and of the New Year." Goddess Gift. Accessed February 25, 2022. https://www.goddessgift.com/goddess-info/meet-the-goddesses/yemaya/yemaya-unabridged/.

GoodTherapy. "Neuro-Linguistic Programming (NLP)." Accessed March 18, 2022. GoodTherapy.org. https://www.goodtherapy.org/learn-about-therapy/types/neuro-linguistic-programming.

Greenberg, Mike. "Who Was the Goddess Hygieia?" Mythology Source. April 26, 2021. https://mythologysource.com/goddess-hygieia/.

Gutierrez, Sam. "Are Your Favorite Candles Slowly Poisoning You?" HouseBeautiful.com. December 26, 2018. https://www.housebeautiful.com/lifestyle/a25656783/candles-bad-for-you/.

Hanson, Neils Viggo; Torben Jørgensen, and Lisbeth Ørtenblad. "Massage and Touch for Dementia." National Center for Biotechnology Information. October 2006. https://www.ncbi.nlm.nih.gov/pmc/articles/PMC6823223/.

Healthline. "How to Safely Get a Massage While Pregnant." Healthline.com. August 27, 2021. https://www.healthline.com/health/pregnancy/where-not-to-massage-a-pregnant-woman#takeaway.

Honey Girl Organics. "15 Toxic Ingredients in Skin Care and Cosmetics Products." HoneyGirlOrganics.com. Accessed March 22, 2022. https://honeygirlorganics.com/pages/15-toxic-ingredients-in-skin-care.

Ingraham, Paul. "Why Drink Water After Massage?" PainScience.com. September 1, 2018. https://www.painscience.com/articles/drinking-water-after-massage.php.

Kothari, Parul, MD. "Epinephrine is the Only Effective Treatment for Anaphylaxis." Harvard Health Publishing/Harvard Medical School. July 9, 2020. https://www.health.harvard.edu/blog/epinephrine-is-the-only-effective-treatment-for-anaphylaxis-2020070920523.

Link, Rachel. "6 Science-Based Health Benefits of Oregano." Healthline.com. October 27, 2017. https://www.healthline.com/nutrition/6-oregano-benefits.

Mark, Joshua. "Tara." August 9, 2021. World History Encyclopedia. https://www.worldhistory.org/Tara_(Goddess)/.

Mayo Clinic Staff. "Massage: Get in Touch With its Many Benefits." Mayo Clinic. January 12, 2021. https://www.mayoclinic.org/healthy-lifestyle/stress-management/in-depth/massage/art-20045743.

Medical Massage Therapy. "Varicose Veins Massage." MassageTherapyReference.com. Accessed July 22, 2022. https://www.massagetherapyreference.com/varicose-veins-massage/.

Medical News Today. "Hugs and Kisses: The Health Impact of Affective Touch." Medical News Today. Accessed October 20, 2021. https://www.medicalnewstoday.com/articles/323143.

Merrill, Claudia. "Airmed, the Celtic Goddess of Healing." ClaudiaMerrill.com. January 8, 2021. https://www.claudiamerrill.com/blog/the-irish-goddess-airmed.

Mount Sinai. "Therapeutic Touch." Mount Sinai. Accessed October 21, 2021. https://www.mountsinai.org/health-library/treatment/therapeutic-touch.

Nagdeve, Meenakshi. "16 Surprising Benefits of Clove Oil." OrganicFacts.net. June 1, 2021. https://www.organicfacts.net/health-benefits/essential-oils/health-benefits-of-clove-oil.html.

National Center for Complementary and Integrative Health. "Massage Therapy for Health: What the Science Says." November 2018. https://www.nccih.nih.gov/health/providers/digest/massage-therapy-for-health-science.

National Center for Complementary and Integrative Health. "Massage Therapy: What You Need to Know." April 2019. https://www.nccih.nih.gov/health/massage-therapy-what-you-need-to-know.

Newman, Mindy. "Embodying the Healing Mother." Fall, 2021; accessed February 26, 2022. Tricycle—The Buddhist Review. https://tricycle.org/magazine/mother-tara-practice/.

Newton, Aline. "Neuroscience of Touch: Touch and the Brain." Aline Newton Rolfing Structural Integration. December 16, 2014. http://alinenewton.com/neuroscience-of-touch-touch-and-the-brain/.

Nordqvist, Joseph. "What are the Health Benefits and Risks of Lavender?" MedicalNews-Today.com. March 4, 2019. https://www.medicalnewstoday.com/articles/265922.

PNSG. "Where NOT to Massage During Pregnancy." March 18, 2020. https://pnsingapore.com/blog/where-not-to-massage-during-pregnancy/.

Physiopedia. "Vagus Nerve." Physiopedia.com. Accessed July 16, 2022. https://www.physio-pedia.com/Vagus_Nerve.

Purhoit, Temple. "Lord Krishna—Hindu Gods and Deities." TemplePurohit.org. Accessed February 25, 2022. https://www.templepurohit.com/hindu-gods-and-deities/lord-krishna/.

Raypole, Crystal. "Touch Therapy: Is It Worth Trying?" Healthline. Accessed October 20, 2021. https://www.healthline.com/health/touch-therapy.

Regina-Whitely, Michael. "Autism and Treatment with Therapeutic Massage." Massage Today. May 29, 2009. https://www.massagetoday.com/articles/13157/Autism-and-Treatment-With-Therapeutic-Massage.

Regula, deTraci. "Selene, Greek Goddess of the Moon." June 26, 2019. ThoughtCo. https://www.thoughtco.com/greek-mythology-selene-1526204.

Rosa, Linda; Rosa, Emily; Sarner, Larry; et al. "A Closer Look at Therapeutic Touch." April 1, 1998. Journal of the American Medical Association (JAMA). https://jamanetwork.com/journals/jama/fullarticle/187390.

Scientific American. "What Makes the Sound When We Crack Our Knuckles?" ScientificAmerican.com. October 26, 2001. https://www.scientificamerican.com/article/what-makes-the-sound-when/.

Shryer, Donna. "Breaking Through: Massage + Autism." American Massage Therapy Association. February 15, 2017. https://www.amtamassage.org/publications /massage-therapy-journal/massage-and-autism/.

Silver, Natalie. "The Benefits of Geriatric Massage." Healthline. May 18, 2021. https:// www.healthline.com/health/geriatric-massage.

Telis, Gisela. "Massage's Mystery Mechanism Unmasked." Science.org. February 1, 2012. https://www.science.org/content/article/massages-mystery-mechanism-unmasked.

The Conversation. "Could Consciousness All Come Down to the Way Things Vibrate?" November 9, 2018. TheConversation.com. https://theconversation.com /could-consciousness-all-come-down-to-the-way-things-vibrate-103070.

Trudeau, Michelle. "Human Connections Start With A Friendly Touch." NPR. September 20, 2010. https://www.npr.org/templates/story/story.php?storyId=128795325.

Twin Rocks Trading Post. "Navajo Changing Woman." Twinrocks.com. Accessed July 16, 2022. https://twinrocks.com/legends/dieties/navajo-changing-woman.html.

University of Colorado at Boulder. "When Lovers Touch, Their Breathing, Heartbeat Syncs, Pain Wanes, Study Shows. ScienceDaily. June 21, 2017. https://www .sciencedaily.com/releases/2017/06/170621125313.htm.

Vallet, Michelle. "A Touch of Compassion: Massage Therapy and Alzheimer's Disease." American Massage Therapy Association. November 15, 2011. https://www .amtamassage.org/publications/massage-therapy-journal/massage-and-alzheimers/.

Vein & Vascular Institute, Editor. "Does Massage Help Varicose Veins." Vein & Vascular Institute. January 15, 2020. https://www.veinvascular.com/vein /does-massage-help-varicose-veins/.

Walla, Nona. "Why You Need a Daily Massage." ETimes/Times of India.com. March 10, 2019. https://timesofindia.indiatimes.com/life-style/health-fitness/de-stress /why-you-need-a-daily-massage/articleshow/68317790.cms.

Warner, Jennifer. "When is an Allergic Reaction an Emergency?" EverydayHealth.com. April 15, 2014. https://www.everydayhealth.com/hs /anaphylaxis-severe-allergy-guide/allergic-reaction-emergency/.

WebMD Editorial Contributors. "Are There Health Benefits to Using Sage Oil?" WebMD. com. October 22, 2020. https://www.webmd.com/diet/health-benefits-sage-oil.

WebMD Editorial Contributors. "Health Benefits of Rosemary." WebMD.com. September 18, 2020. https://www.webmd.com/diet/health-benefits-rosemary.

Weizmann Institute of Science. "Quantum Theory Demonstrated: Observation Affects Reality." Science Daily. February 26, 1998. https://www.sciencedaily.com/releases/1998/02/980227055013.htm.

Wigington, Patti. "Gods and Goddesses of Healing." Learn Religions. April 26, 2019. https://www.learnreligions.com/gods-and-goddesses-of-healing-2561980.

Ydalir. "Norse Gods: Eir." Ydalir.ca. Accessed February 25, 2022. http://ydalir.ca/norsegods/eir/.

Zinti, Amy. "How to Massage a Baby." Parents.com. October 3, 2005. https://www.parents.com/baby/care/newborn/how-to-massage-baby/.

To Write to the Author

If you wish to contact the author or would like more information about this book, please write to the author in care of Llewellyn Worldwide Ltd. and we will forward your request. Both the author and the publisher appreciate hearing from you and learning of your enjoyment of this book and how it has helped you. Llewellyn Worldwide Ltd. cannot guarantee that every letter written to the author can be answered, but all will be forwarded. Please write to:

Debra DeAngelo
⁒ Llewellyn Worldwide
2143 Wooddale Drive
Woodbury, MN 55125-2989

Please enclose a self-addressed stamped envelope for reply, or $1.00 to cover costs. If outside the U.S.A., enclose an international postal reply coupon.

Many of Llewellyn's authors have websites with additional information and resources. For more information, please visit our website at http://www.llewellyn.com